THE

SUNSET
YEARS

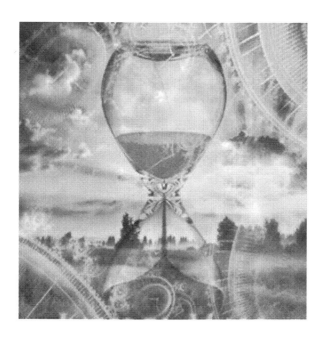

Aging: Issues & Concerns

LAUREL HALL

LAUREL HALL

Other books by this author:

Providence
Expressions
Betrayed

LCCN: 2013920057

ISBN-13: 978-1492747109
ISBN-10: 1492747106

Printed in the United States of America

THE SUNSET YEARS

For

Dr. Jack

Acknowledgements

- Special acknowledgement to Gloria Starling with Terra Nova Films for allowing me to use excerpts in this book from several of their films.

- To Lucy Alexander for giving me permission to quote a sentence from her article, An Ethical Perspective on Institutional Abuse of Older Adults. **Garner, J. and Evans, S. (2002)** The Psychiatrist 26, 164-166) Lucy Alexander.

- To Karin Cox, special friend, mentor, and great teacher, you are terrific. Special thanks and appreciation to you.

- To my friendly readers, thank you for giving of your time to read the manuscript. I am grateful to you for your comments and insights.

- Special thanks to my editor, Mike Valentino, and to Robert Kauffman for the cover design and his assistance with the interior layout.

- Thanks to my husband and family for their support and for sharing their thoughts, ideas, and other information on aging.

THE SUNSET YEARS

Authors Quoted

- Butler, Samuel (1835–1902) English author
- Carter, Jimmy (1924–Present) James Earl
  Carter, Jr. 39th President of the United States
- Coleridge, Samuel Taylor (1771-1834) English
  poet, literary critic and philosopher.
- Cowper, William (1731-1800) English poet
- Emerson, Ralph Waldo (1803-1881) American essayist
  Lecturer, poet
- Feltham, Owen (1602-1668) English writer and author
- Gay, John (1685-1732) English poet and dramatist
- Keats, John (1795-1821) English poet
- Plautus, Titus Maccius (254-184 BC)
  Best known comic Roman playwright
- Rowe, Nicholas (1674-1747) Poet Laureate,
  Samuel Johnson called Rowe's translation of
  Lucan "one of the greatest productions of
  English poetry".
- Scott, Sir Walter (1771-1832) Scottish historical
  novelist, playwright, poet
- Shakespeare, William (1564-1616) English poet and playwright

LAUREL HALL

THE SUNSET YEARS

Author's Introduction

I really did not want to write another book. Having just completed *Betrayed,* I was worn-out. I gave the first copy of the book to a friend, who is also a medical doctor. After reading it he said: *"I wish you had written something on elder abuse. That is a huge group that I encounter in my daily practice."* Being unfamiliar with elder abuse, I decided to look into it as a future book. Researching the topic was incredibly disheartening. No one would want to read solely about the abuse some seniors endured. It would be too depressing. I decided to change the format to include other issues and concerns faced by the elderly including dementia, Alzheimer's disease, and more. Then the question entered my mind: *What can people do to have a* healthier and happier sunset? That needed to be addressed as well.

So, here it is. It is my hope you find this information useful in your life's journey. Let me also say, this book was not intended to be an in-depth study, but rather a snapshot of the issues and concerns of aging. Sources and references have been included at the end for further reading. LH

LAUREL HALL

THE SUNSET YEARS

Table of Contents

LAUREL HALL

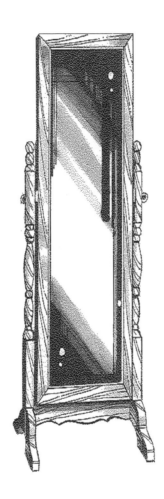

THE SUNSET YEARS

Reflection

I look in the mirror
and what do I see?
I don' t see the girl
I used to be.
I see a woman
with sagging skin;
not really fat,
definitely not thin.
I'd like to be younger,
but not really young;
I like the person
I have become.
But yet, somehow
inside of me,
I think myself young
as I used to be.

From Expressions
By Laurel Hall, 2012

LAUREL HALL

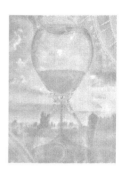

Make the most of yourself
for that's all there is of you.
Ralph Waldo Emerson

Chapter One
Overview

I t was a cold January day. The storm had been raging for several hours and the wind was now blowing the snow in drifts. Emma was sitting by the fireplace in her favorite brown leather recliner with her legs up. She felt so relaxed, savoring the moment when Jon came in with the mail.

"Here's a letter for you from the hospital."

"Wonder what they want"? She opened the letter and began to read.

Dear Ms. Johnson,

As a hospital we are frequently providing our employees with continuing education to keep them current on medical topics. We are planning a seminar on issues and concerns of our elderly population. We have prepared a syllabus and have enclosed it for you to review. We would like to interview you for the teaching position. We are aware of your teaching skills and the books you have written on abuse. Would you be interested in conducting the class? Our staff feels you would be the perfect candidate. If you are interested please call us to set up an interview within two weeks.

Jon ran his fingers through his hair. "That would entail a lot of preparation. How do you feel about that?"

"I have to think about it." Emma held the letter in her hands, wondering how she would teach such a class. She hadn't taught in years, and when she did, her classes were high school students. This would be totally different. Her students would be nurses, medical students doing their internship, technicians, nurse practitioners, physician assistants, and doctors. She was well aware of the amount of time it would take to prepare to teach this class. She would have to educate herself on the concerns of elders, dementia and Alzheimer's disease, the various types of elder abuse, and the laws dealing with elder abuse. Most people have heard of Alzheimer's disease and dementia, but elder abuse is not a common topic of conversation. How to present the course of study was another matter. Perhaps she might break the classes up with abuse and another topic. Perhaps she would use a 'h a n d s - o n' style of teaching where the students present as well. Maybe she would use guest speakers. All these thoughts circled through her mind.

The next day she called the hospital to set up an interview. It went well. They presented her with a course outline including all the topics they would like her to cover during the seminar.

THE SUNSET YEARS

The class would not begin until mid-June giving her three months to prepare. After discussing it with Jon, Emma decided to take the assignment.

First, she chose to learn about elder abuse and was dismayed with what she discovered. Although most seniors and elderly were enjoying a good life, for some it was pure misery. The importance of solid family relationships became all too evident. Emma was lucky that she had a wonderful family who would watch after her as she aged and she felt certain that they would never abuse her.

She then studied what issues and concerns seniors have in general. As the body ages and grows weak, elders become afraid of falling and perhaps breaking a hip or leg. Also, as their friends die, loneliness becomes an issue.

Dementia and Alzheimer's were next on her list. Here she learned that some forms of dementia were reversible, but most were not. She discovered there were two different types of Alzheimer's disease, one genetic, one not. The more she studied she found herself becoming depressed with the situation of the elderly, particularly the tragedy of elder abuse. She found a website, Terra Nova Films, which specialized in movies and videos dealing with problems some older people face. Some were difficult to watch, but they would be another tool to use in the class.

Emma spent hours each day reviewing the subject matter and after nine weeks of preparation she felt ready to teach the class.

The ringing phone startled her. "Emma, this is Marcie Withers, the hospital coordinator for education. I wanted to check in with you about the seminar you will be presenting. Will you be ready to begin teaching in three weeks?"

"I will" Emma replied. "I have just about completed

preparation for the class and am eagerly looking forward to presenting it."

"That's good news. We are anticipating forty students. Class will be held in a large conference room on the sixth floor of the hospital. Are Wednesday mornings from 7-9 a.m. a good time for you?"

"Yes, that will be fine."

"Great. We will see you then. Good bye, Emma."

Putting down the phone, Emma turned to Jon.

"I must say I feel a bit intimidated. The students probably know more than I do. Am I competent to teach this class? There are going to be doctors listening to me, a lay person, speak!"

"They're people just like you, and they want to know what you have learned. You were a terrific math teacher, and received outstanding scores in your teaching skills. You're going to do great. "

Emma smiled. Jon always knew the right thing to say. He was her biggest cheerleader.

*****

The day for class had finally come. Today it was going to be hot! *This is really unusual for June, but I'm glad I'm not in Houston,* Emma thought as she walked from her car to the building. She and Jon had lived in Houston some forty years, and she was well familiar with the weather in that part of the country. *In addition to being hot it would be unbearably muggy. At least here in Colorado the humidity is fairly low.* A pleasant breeze contributed to making the walk more comfortable.

Emma had dressed in blue slacks with a blue and white three-quarter length cotton shirt. She added a long blue and silver necklace along with silver earrings, and a pair of blue sandals to complete her outfit. Her hair was cut short in a pixie style hairdo with a few curls on top. On a recent trip to California she had purchased a pair of "professional looking" eyeglasses which she felt made her look more qualified for the role. All this to build up her confidence to speak to such an esteemed group.

As she entered the building the cool air-conditioned air was a welcome relief. A woman, probably in her mid-forties came up to her, extending her hand.

"Are you Emma Johnson?"

"Yes," Emma replied.

"My name is Marcie Withers. I'm with the hospital and will introduce you to your class. We have a number of students eager to learn about the problems of aging."

Emma smiled. "Hi Marcie. It's so good to finally meet you after talking with you on the telephone."

"We are excited to have you here to teach this class. Would you like to go to the conference room where class will be held, or have a cup of coffee first?"

"I think I would like to see where I will be teaching." The room was on the top floor of the building, large, open, and airy. Two walls were all glass and afforded a spectacular view of the mountains. Room darkening shades had been provided to be used if needed as well as a pull down screen to show video material. At the front of the room was a podium. Someone had placed a bottle of water along with a paper cup there for her. The remaining walls were painted a pale silver blue. The tables were round and could seat up to eight students each in comfortable looking, padded leather folding chairs.

"Oh, this is perfect!" exclaimed Emma. "I was hoping the students could be seated in groups. I plan to use a 'hands-on' style method of teaching, where the students are totally involved. Was each student given a number from one to eight as I had requested?"

"Oh, yes," Marcie said and smiled. "They wondered about the purpose of those numbers."

"I like to group students that perhaps do not know each other, have different skills, and such. I brought numbers to put on each table, and students with that number will all sit together at the table with the same number."

"Hmm. Sounds interesting," said Marcie. "That way all the doctors don't sit together, all the nurses, etc."

"Right" Emma replied. "Students will get to know each other and will be able to interact on a personal level alongside those with different abilities and positions. I've used it in the past. Here's hoping I get the same results here."

"We have a few minutes before class starts. Would you like to go get a cup of coffee?" asked Marcie.

"No thank you, Marcie. I think I would just as soon stay here and get organized and greet the students as they arrive."

"Good idea. I'll be back shortly."

Emma looked around the room. *This is perfect*, she thought. She had never held class in such posh surroundings. A table with ice water, coffee and a few cookies and pastries had been provided for the students. Walking around the room she placed a piece of paper with a number on each of the tables as well as a stack of booklets. She removed the notes she had on elder abuse from her briefcase and put them on the podium. She planned to discuss abuse with the class in-depth, but today would only be an overview of the issue. Each type of abuse would be discussed in detail later. Turning around, she stood there looking out at the empty chairs that would soon be occupied. Emma felt the teacher in her return as her heart swelled with excitement. She was ready!

THE SUNSET YEARS

Learning by study must be won;
T'was néer entail'd from sire to son.

John Gay

Chapter Two
The Students

T he time passed quickly and soon men and women of
all ages were flowing into the room. Some were nurses
dressed in colorful tops and coordinating blue bottoms.
Others were apparently doctors wearing white coats
with a stethoscope around their neck. Two were dressed in
green, as if ready for surgery. Emma was standing at the door
to greet them all, asking them what their number was and
helping them to find their table. Everyone seemed happy and
quickly found their places.

Within moments Marcie entered the room. After the

students were seated she and Emma walked to the front of the room. "Good morning. We are glad each of you took the opportunity to attend this class. Hopefully at the end of the sessions we will know more about issues and concerns of the elderly than we do today. Classes will meet once a week, in this same location, every Wednesday at 7 – 9 a.m. for eight weeks. We are fortunate to have Emma Johnson as our teacher. She is a former educator and author having written on child abuse. Please give her a warm Colorado welcome."

Marcie slowly moved to the back of the room and took a seat. As the students applauded, Emma moved to the podium. "Thank you, Marcie. It is an honor for me to be here today to share with all of you what I have learned on the many issues of aging. During our time together we will discuss the challenges and fears of senior citizens, the diseases of dementia and Alzheimer's, elder abuse, laws designed to protect seniors, and more."

"I have seated you in groups and the people at your table will be your teammates. On each table there is a piece of paper with a number on it. That is your group number. If you will turn the paper over you will find a specific category of elder abuse. That is the assignment for the people seated at that table. It is my hope everyone in the group will work together to prepare a presentation on that particular type of elder abuse and present it to the class. I have also placed a workbook for each of you on your table. As you prepare for your discussion on the topic you have been given, read through the workbook and be certain you have covered all the questions presented in it."

"Before we begin I would like for each of you to introduce yourselves to each of the members of your group." The room became a bit noisy as each person introduced themselves to the group and began to discuss the topic of discussion.

After five minutes or so Emma asked, "Which group has "Physical abuse?""

Group Two raised their hands.

"Would you introduce yourselves and then share with us what you know about physical abuse." As they did this Emma drew a circle and wrote the name of the students as they were given and the group number.

A beautiful young woman with chestnut colored hair stood up first. "My name is Rebecca Rodriquez. I'm a surgical nurse. This is my third year with this hospital. Although I know it exists, I am really not familiar with elder abuse."

Next, a middle-aged man stood up. "My name is Gary Friend. I work in the MRI department. I've been with the hospital six years. I know a little about child abuse, but very little about elder abuse, although I imagine it might be similar."

A young woman with sandy blonde hair and a fair complexion stood next. "My name is Sharon Linn. I am a registered nurse and work in a doctor's office. I have not studied elder abuse."

Next, a tall, slender man arose. He had an air of self-confidence and piercing blue eyes. Emma looked at him and smiled. He had operated on her friend, Holly, when she had needed surgery some years back. "My name is John Arthur. I am a surgeon at this hospital. Although I am familiar with elder abuse, I am far from being an expert."

He continued. "As a group we agreed physical abuse includes bodily harm or more to an elderly person."

"Thank you for your introductions. It's a pleasure to have

each of you in class. You are correct," Emma added. "Physical abuse includes any kind of bodily injury to an elder by an abuser. Some signs of physical abuse can be more elusive, such as restraint marks on the elder's wrist or broken eyeglasses. Thank you."

In her notes she wrote Group Two, physical abuse; Rebecca, surgical nurse; Gary, MRI; Sharon, RN; John, surgeon.

"Which group has Emotional/Verbal abuse?" Group Four raised their hands.

"Great. Would you each introduce yourselves and then share what you know about Emotional/Verbal abuse."

The first to stand was a young Asian man in his mid-twenties. "My name is Hai Wong. I am a nurse and have been working here at the hospital for two years. I know a little about elder abuse, but have not studied it per se."

"My name is Marion Mahoney," a woman in her early fifties said as she stood up. "I am an anesthesiologist and work both here and at another hospital in town. I have read some on abuse, particularly child abuse, but very little on elder abuse."

An older woman stood. "My name is Susan Bonds and I've been a nurse for thirty years. I work in obstetrics. I am somewhat familiar with child abuse, but not elder abuse."

A young girl stood next. She was obviously very nervous as she spoke. "My name is Lucy Rose. I work in the lab. I draw blood," she said laughingly. "I really know nothing about abuse."

A young woman in her mid-thirties was next. "My name is Jennifer Thomas. I am a doctor in the field of internal medicine. We decided verbal abuse is speaking to another in a way which humiliates, perhaps by making fun of them in a cruel manner."

"Thank you and it's a pleasure to meet you. You are right. Verbal abuse does include humiliating, ridiculing, or constantly criticizing another. It is a form of emotional abuse and can also be non-verbal. Good job." Once more in her notes she had written Group Four, verbal; Hai, nurse; Mahoney, anesthesiologist; Susan, obstetrics nurse; Lucy, lab; Jen, internal medicine.

"Which group has Financial abuse?" Group Three raised their hands.

Once again they introduced themselves as Emma took notes. In Group Three was a pathologist, Dr. Herman Sparks, three nurses, Hugo Gonzales, Muriel Burns, and Maria Delgado, and Dr. Maarten Johansen, an orthopedic surgeon. Dr. Johansen spoke for the group. "We believe financial abuse includes stealing from an elderly person, be it money, jewelry, or whatever."

"Yes" said Emma. "Financial abuse is a more subtle form of abuse and occurs when someone obtains from the elder money, property, jewelry, or other valuables illegally. Many times the abuser is able to do this because he has unlawfully obtained power of attorney over his victim. Sometimes an abuser will deprive the elder of his money, get title to his home, and then may even try to evict him."

"Which group has Sexual abuse?" Group One raised their hands.

As with the other groups they each took turns introducing themselves. The first was Mike Benson, a police officer for the state of Colorado. He was here to check out the class to determine if it should be used again with all the policemen in his precinct. Next was Dr. Robert Holland, a gastroenterologist, Dr. Ricardo Gutierrez, an ER doctor, and two nurses, Barbara Edwards and Sally Calitri. Sally spoke for the group. "We believe sexual abuse is coercing an elder to take part in sexual activity without permission."

"Yes, that is correct. Sexual abuse of an elder includes making him or her take part in any kind of sexual activity without consent, or compelling participation in conversations of a sexual nature against his will. Visible signs on the body, especially around the breasts or genital area, unexplained infections, as well as ripped undergarments can be evidence of such abuse."

"Which group has Neglect?" Group Five raised their hands.

There were five members in Group Five, all nurses: Ann Haver, Mark Kellogg, Judy Kelp, Claire Donahue, and Barbara Kelly. After introductions, Barbara said, "We believe neglect includes such things as not providing food, heat, clothing and such."

"Yes, that is right, Barbara. Neglect can also include depriving medication or necessary services to an elder. Sometimes an elder refuses to care for themselves. That is called self-neglect."

"Good job! Which group has Abandonment?" A hand from Group Seven was raised.

There were five members in that group. Two doctors: Dr. Tom Parsons, a heart specialist and Dr. Jim Howard, a pediatrician; three nurses, Janet Odom, Tim Hollis, and Irma Brown. They each worked in different areas and did not know each other. Dr. Parsons spoke for the group. "As a group we feel abandonment is a type of abuse where the elder is left alone or unattended for a period of time which might put their health and welfare in danger."

"Very good. Abandonment can be either emotional or physical. Thank you for being part of our class. Who has

Institutional abuse?"

All the students in Group Six raised their hands. There were five members: two nurses, Jamie Luciano and Bethany Rolf; one doctor, Dr. Rockey Evans, the hospital doctor; and two x-ray technicians, Jeanne Levine and Sarah Driscoll. Dr. Evans spoke for the group. "We believe institutional abuse includes physical or psychological harm where care and help is provided to the elder in a paid care facility."

"You are absolutely right," said Emma. "It's a pleasure having you in class as well. Group Eight, I assume you have Patients' Rights abuse," Emma said and smiled. "Would you introduce yourselves to the class?"

In that group there were two attorneys, one doctor, and two nurses. As they introduced themselves Emma wrote down their names: Dr. Jacob Webber, hematologist; Betty Cornwall, surgical nurse; Jane Ruth, general nursing; Dale Dobson, civil rights attorney; and Walter Carbonera, attorney of international law. *How perfect*, Emma thought and smiled - *Two attorneys in the rights group*. Attorney James spoke for the group. "Patients' rights abuse is where the individual is denied his rights due to age," he said. Then, he added, "Most people are not familiar with patients' rights."

"That is true," said Emma. "From the answers you have given, I am impressed with your knowledge of elder abuse. This should provide for an interesting class and lively discussions."

"We will be discussing elder abuse in the latter part of the course, but I would like to take this time to make a few comments on the subject. Elder abuse is an 'out of sight' problem and tends to be committed mostly by family members in the privacy of the elder person's home. As with most victims of abuse, whether child, adult, or elder, the victim may not realize he or she is being abused. Abuse is not a word in their vocabulary. All they know is that someone doesn't like them and is treating them badly and they feel trapped. Elderly victims may think this is how it is when you get old and it is entirely their fault. They have done something to cause anger on the part of the abuser. The victim is afraid others won't believe him if he reports what is going on and how he or she is being treated, or is afraid he will be institutionalized. The perpetrator may be the only human interaction the elder has and if he reports on the treatment he is receiving, the offender may retaliate in the future. If the elder is in ill health or has cognitive decline, he/she may be unable to report any kind of maltreatment."

"Older people with memory problems, physical disabilities, depression, loneliness, and substance abuse, including alcohol, are much more susceptible to abuse than others. Sometimes the elderly person is combative with the caregiver and the caregiver feels overwhelmed or offended. Also, if the caregiver is dependent on the older person for housing, finances or other needs, is otherwise unemployed, or perhaps with mental health problems or a criminal history, the chances for elder abuse increase greatly."

"Health officials, in particular doctors, are able to play an important role by reporting elder abuse, but few physicians tend to contact authorities with regards to situations with which they are familiar. There are several reasons for this. Among them are lack of knowledge of state laws, concern with angering the offender, damaging the rapport they have established with the patient, as well as potential appearances in court, lack of collaboration from the victim/patient and/or his family, and lack of time."

"Those employed in the legal system including police, attorneys, and judges need to be instructed on elder abuse. Legislation to protect elderly victims will help to minimize such

THE SUNSET YEARS

abuse and provide help to the injured party. Involvement by the community, creating programs designed to help seniors and meet their needs is essential. These programs would include monetary aid, tax assistance, and help from public and private professionals who would be willing to volunteer their time to help the elderly. I might add elder abuse does not just happen here in the United States. It is a global issue and needs to be addressed."

"I chose a 'hands-on' style to teach abuse because by studying the topic yourselves you will internalize the problems some elderly people face. You will have several weeks to complete your research prior to presentation. In order to be fair, I have put each group number in a bowl. When the time comes I will draw out two numbers and those will be the groups to present the following week. You may use whatever resources you wish including films, case studies and such." Handing out a sheet of paper to each student, Emma said, "Here are a few resources you may use. Feel free to search out the Internet, your local library and more."

Emma took a sip of water and looked at her watch. "Our time is about up. Thank you all for being here and in making this day a success. You have made me feel very welcome."

After all the students had left Marcie walked to the front of the room. "Good job, Emma. I think we found the right teacher."

"Thank you, Marcie. I enjoyed it. I must admit I was a bit daunted at first, but Jon was right, they're all people just like you and me."

As they took the elevator down Marcie asked, "Do you mind if I continue in the course as a group member?"

"That would be great, Marcie. Group Two has only four members, sit with them next week."

"I will. Thank you."

As Emma walked to her car she felt good inside. The class, she sensed, had been a success. As she drove home she stopped to pick up a latte. She couldn't wait to tell Jon about her morning.

*****

Jon was waiting when Emma arrived home. "How did it go?"

"It went great! There are 40 students in the class including Dr. Arthur. He was my friend Holly's surgeon a number of years back. Do you remember him?

" Yes. Holly thought he was an excellent doctor."

" She did. The one thing she liked about him was that he was such a gentleman. I remember she had said some doctors are rather abrupt, not seemingly interested in their patient as a person. Dr. Arthur wasn't that way."

"Well, how were the students?" asked Jon.

" The students made me feel comfortable and welcome. And the room! You should see it, Jon. Two walls are all glass with a magnificent view of the mountains. Round tables with padded leather folding chairs for the students - it was really nice! The hospital had provided refreshments for the break, and they were gone before the end of class," Emma said laughingly.

"And were you intimidated?"

"Oh, maybe a little at first, but everyone made me feel so welcome, I was at ease in no time."

"I knew you could do it. Congratulations."

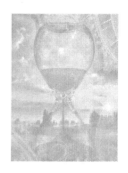

"Age sits with decent grace upon his visage,
And worthily becomes his silver locks;
He bears the marks of many years well-spent,
A virtuous truth well tried,
and wise experience."

N. Rowe

Chapter Three
Senior Issues

E mma spent a good part of the week trying to learn the names of her students, their positions with the hospital and such. She had made a class roster naming each group by number along with the topic for which they were respons- ible. She would place one for each person at every table hoping it would help the students in becoming acquainted with each other. When Wednesday came Emma arrived at the hospital early and once there took the elevator to the sixth floor. No one had arrived yet. She placed the rosters on each table, took out her notes and was looking over them as the students began to arrive. A number of students started to gather around Emma. They looked like they wanted to say something. Finally, Rebecca from Group Two spoke up: "We just want you to know we are looking forward to these classes. We think you will be a wonderful teacher."

"Thank you. You are a remarkable group of students and I know I will enjoy being your instructor."

"We feel fortunate to have you to present this material," said Marcie.

"You make me feel so special. Thank you." As they returned to their seats, the rest of the students began to arrive. Soon the classroom was filled. Emma began. "Good morning all. On your table I have placed a class roster for each of you to help you become familiar with your classmates." As the students picked them up, she continued. "Today our discussion will be on issues affecting the health and welfare of seniors." Picking up her class roster she asked Rockey Evans, the hospital doctor: "Dr. Evans, in your day to day practice what do you think is the most serious issue affecting the health of the elderly?"

"I don't know if it's the most serious issue, but I think perhaps loneliness is an issue."

"I think you are right. When seniors begin surviving their friends and relatives, they usually become depressed and lonely. People they have known for many years, sometimes over their lifetime, are gone. If they have no children or no children living nearby to visit them on a regular basis, and/or have no friends left to stopover once in a while, it can be devastating. Humans thrive on friendship, support, kindness and the caring of others. Even though they may have the TV on all day, it does not replace human contact. Having a loving, supportive family near to visit and to have conversation is truly a blessing. Any comments?" Emma asked.

Judy Kelp, one of the nurses in Group Five raised her hand. "When I was a child, maybe ten years old, I asked my uncle who was maybe seventy, but old to me, if he minded growing old and if he was afraid of dying. He said, '*no, all my friends are gone, and even though I have family, it's not the same.*' I looked at him and smiled, continuing doing whatever it was."

"Thank you, Judy, for sharing that."

"Dr. Webber, can you think of another issue concerning the elderly?"

"I have an elderly aunt and she has told me several times she is afraid of falling."

"That is a concern," replied Emma. "Seniors who have had health issues, such as strokes, brain injuries, and poor vision, foot and leg problems are constantly afraid of falling. My own mother had no fluid in her knees and when she walked it was bone on bone and very painful. She would have been a good candidate for a knee replacement surgery, but she waited too long. At ninety the doctors felt she was too old to undergo the operation. We had fluid injected in her knees which helped, but it was still painful for her to walk. Unfortunately, for many seniors, some falls are too big for their body to recover from and may be the beginning of an irreversible health decline."

"Dr. Johansen, can you think of another concern?"

"I think another concern might be diet — are they getting the proper nutrition and enough liquids, especially water."

"Yes. Seniors tend to neglect themselves if there is no

one around to cook for them. They are likely to eat things they can cook quickly, but might not be good for them on a regular basis. They probably eat few fresh fruits and vegetables, and very few are likely to spend time preparing a healthy, good tasting meal just for themselves. When a person is dealing with pain, memory loss, or chronic disabilities, they want to keep things simple."

Dr. Evans raised his hand. "We see in the emergency room many seniors admitted for dehydration. They neglect themselves by not drinking enough fluids that their bodies require and then wind up in the hospital."

"Yes", Emma replied. "Seniors living around people who care about them usually don't usually have this problem. They are the lucky ones."

"What might be another concern," Emma asked of the class.

Janet Odom, a nurse from Group Seven, raised her hand. "I think taking medicines might be an issue."

"Very good, Janet," Emma answered. "Many times seniors do not take their medicines on time or can't remember what and how much to take. Often seniors take a lot of different medicines, some before meals, some with meals, and some at bedtime. It can get confusing. Many times seniors forget where they put their pills, or how many they should take."

Hai Wong from Group Four raised his hand. "One of the things we did for my grandmother was to buy a 'pill minder' for medications. She lived with us and my parents would put her medicines in this contraption, and then when it was time to take the pills an alarm went off. It worked well. It helped my mother, too, because when she heard the alarm, she knew it was pill time."

"That's a good idea," said Emma. "Do you know where

they purchased it?"

"I believe it was on Amazon," Hai replied.

"Thank you, Hai, for sharing that information. Who can think of another concern?" asked Emma.

Dr. Thomas, from Group Four, spoke. "I think exercise might be a problem. I believe at some point seniors give up, thinking nothing they do is going to help them improve and they stop trying."

"I believe that is so" said Emma. "Exercise is probably one of the most important things an elderly person can do. Exercise has many positive benefits: It can help control weight, lower blood pressure, strengthens muscles, improves circulation, increases appetite and allows them to sleep more restfully. Stretching is also very important. As we age our muscles tend to shorten and get stiff. Just five minutes of stretching will help improve flexibility."

"What can we as families do to help our elderly relatives, parents, and friends feel worthwhile, not forgotten?" asked Emma.

Sarah Driscoll raised her hand. "One thing we can do is devote some of our time with them. Going out to eat together, perhaps taking them to a movie, or just sitting around and visiting with them would make them feel wanted".

"Good answer, Sarah." Bethany, who was sitting next to Sarah, added: "If the elderly person is a relative have them tell you about their life, their parents, aunts, uncles, and so on. How did they celebrate Christmas? Thanksgiving? Was it a big deal in their home?"

Hugo Gonzales raised his hand. "Maybe you can create a family tree, with photographs, having them tell you details about your relatives that you might not know. What kind of work did his/her father do? Did the mother work outside the home? Have talks about siblings, what line of work were they in? How about their education? Does the elder remember her grandparents? What were their names? What did they do for a living? Where were they from? Maybe one came over on the Mayflower."

"All good ideas, Hugo."

Dr. Parsons raised his hand and added: "Another thing you might want to do is create a medical history. Find out what diseases run in your family. Was diabetes in your family? Cancer? Dementia? If you have children or grandchildren get them involved. Get them excited about genealogy."

"That's a great idea" said Emma.

Sharon Linn raised her hand. "If the senior is in a wheelchair, offer to take them outside for a ride on the sidewalk. Try to visit them regularly. Give them something to look forward to as well as giving their caregiver a break."

"Very good idea, Sharon". Then Emma added: "All people want to feel loved. Hug them and let them know you love and care about them, how they feel, and so on. Let them tell you if they hurt and what their concerns are. Listen. Don't cut them off. I believe if we make the elderly part of our lives, it will help with most of these issues, especially loneliness."

"Are there any questions or comments?" There were none. "Good discussion, all. Let's take a short break and when we come back we will discuss dementia."

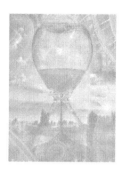

*"Last scene of all
That ends this strange eventful history,
Is second childishness, and mere oblivion;
Sans teeth, sans eyes, sans taste,
Sans everything."*
Shakespeare

Chapter Four
Dementia

After all the students were reseated, Emma stepped to the front of the room. "Dementia is a condition some of the elderly face and needs to be included in any discussion on the problems the elderly face.   Later on we will also discuss Alzheimer's disease. Let me be clear, I am by no means an expert on either dementia or Alzheimer's disease. Having read and studied these conditions I will share with you what I have learned. Perhaps some of you will be willing to add something as well. Before beginning, allow me to ease your minds. Just because you can't find your car keys does not mean you have dementia or Alzheimer's. If you don't recall what the keys are for, well that might indicate a problem." The class laughed.

"Many elderly people have a slight loss of recent memory that doesn't affect their daily functioning. This is called 'mild cognitive impairment'. It does not necessarily mean they have dementia, but it *could* be the early stages of the disease. Some stay at this stage for a long time".

"Does anyone know where the word 'dementia' comes from?"

Dr. Parsons from Group Seven raised his hand. "I believe it comes from the Latin, but I'm not for certain."

"It does come from the Latin. The word 'de' meaning without, and 'ment' meaning 'mind' gives us the word dementia, which we define as a loss of brain function that occurs with certain diseases. It is the loss of conscious intellectual activity such as thinking, reasoning, or remembering. " What causes dementia?" she asked and then answered. " The main risk factor is aging, but as you will soon learn, there are many causes of dementia."

"Who can give me some warning signs of dementia?"

Emma looked around and saw a hand go up.

"Yes, Marcie"?

"I guess when a person begins to lose his memory, or has difficulty with day to day activities, would be a sign."

"Very good. Signs of dementia can vary depending on what is causing the problem and the area of the brain that is affected.

- Memory loss is the initial and most visible indication. The person has problems remembering recent events or recognizing people and places.
- Difficulty finding the right words.
- Difficulty with organizational types of activities, such as writing a letter, or following a recipe.
- Not knowing what to do in an emergency.
- Mood swings. Depression is common and anxiety or hostility may also be present.
- Self-neglect, not wanting to bathe or take care of themselves."

"Are all dementias the same? Anyone? Yes, Hai?"

"I have read that all dementias are not the same, but I am not familiar with the different names they have. I believe they are caused by different things."

"Yes, you are right, Hai. There are various forms of dementia. One type is known as Lewy Body Dementia. Lewy bodies are irregular minute protein build-ups that develop in the interior of nerve cells disturbing the brain's normal operations causing it to slowly deteriorate. Loss of reasoning, mental abilities or motor control is common with people with Lewy body dementia. They often have very vivid fantasies or hallucinations, and may fall frequently."

Does anyone know of another type of dementia? Yes, Marion."

Dr. Mahoney stood as she began to speak. "Another type is called Frontotemporal Dementia, a condition resulting from the gradual deterioration of the frontal lobe of the brain. The first symptoms of this form of dementia may be behavioral changes or strange conduct, inability to express feelings for others. These patients may be rude or impolite and might expose themselves or make blatant sexually explicit remarks."

"Thank you for that information, Dr. Mahoney." Even though Marion was an anesthesiologist she was quite familiar with Alzheimer's. Apparently, an aunt and uncle both suffered from it and she had studied it extensively to learn what she could do to prevent herself from getting the disease.

"Are there some kinds of dementia that comes on rapidly?" asked Jamie Luciano from Group Six.

"Yes, there are," answered Emma. "Sometimes dementia appears suddenly. When it does it might suggest Vascular Dementia, a condition where the blood supply to the brain becomes obstructed. Such a disorder is usually caused by a series of minor strokes. It is the second most common form of dementia after Alzheimer's disease. According to one reference, Vascular Dementia is preventable; therefore, early detection and an accurate diagnosis are important."

Dr. Arthur raised his hand. "There is another quick onset of dementia caused by delirium, a condition which might be the result of a new or worsening illness. Taking away alcohol or drugs, chemical disorders in the body, surgery, toxins, and bacterial infections such as pneumonia and/or urinary tract infections may also bring this on. However, it is more likely in people who already have some brain damage from a stroke or dementia."

"Thank you, Dr. Arthur."

"If a person has memory loss does that mean he has dementia?" asked Emma. "Anyone?"

"I hope not," Dr. Webber said as he stood. "Just because a person has memory loss does not indicate dementia. Conditions such as depression can be treated and do not indicate dementia. Also, problems that come with aging such as forgetting someone's name are not signs of dementia."

"Well," said Emma, "what causes dementia?"

Dr. Garcia stood up. "Dementia is caused by injury to or changes in the brain. Alzheimer's disease is the most common cause of dementia followed by stroke."

"Can dementia be reversed?" asked Emma to the class. "Let's do a show of hands. How many believe dementia can be reversed?" About ten hands were raised. "How many believe it cannot be reversed?" About ten more hands were raised. "How many don't know?" About half the class raised their hands.

"Believe it or not," said Emma, "some causes of dementia can be reversed with treatment, but most cannot. When dementia is caused by curable problems, the treatment may also help the dementia."

Emma raised the paper on the large chart in front of the room. "These are the problems that can cause dementia which can be treated. I started taking B12 today, just in case," she said smiling.

1. Hypothyroidism
2. Vitamin B12 deficiency
3. Lead poisoning
4. Medicines or drug interactions
5. Some brain tumors
6. Normal-pressure hydrocephalus (a condition in which the fluid around the brain is not properly absorbed and adversely affects brain function.)
7. Some cases of chronic alcoholism
8. Some cases of irritation and swelling of the brain, most often due to infection (Encephalitis)
9. HIV/AIDS.

Then she flipped the page over. "The following cases of dementia cannot be reversed. I was unaware that so many diseases caused dementia," she added.

1. Parkinson's disease
2. Dementia with Lewy bodies.
3. Frontotemporal Dementia
4. Pick's disease (a rare illness that causes gradual destruction of nerve cells in the brain.)
5. Severe head injury resulting in a loss of consciousness
6. Vascular Dementia that may occur in people who have a stroke, long-term high blood pressure, or severe hardening of the arteries (atherosclerosis).
7. Huntington's disease (a disorder passed down through families in which nerve cells in certain parts of the brain waste away, or degenerate.)
8. Leukoencephalopathies (a rare and fatal viral diseases that affects the deeper, white-matter brain tissue.)
9. Creutzfeldt-Jakob (a degenerative neurological disorder, a rare and fatal condition that destroys brain tissue. It is sometimes called the human form of 'Mad Cow Disease'.)
10. Brain injuries from accidents or sports activities.
11. Some cases of multiple sclerosis (MS) or amyotrophic lateral sclerosis (ALS), also known as Lou Gehrig's disease
12. Multiple-system degeneration (brain diseases affecting speech, movement, and autonomic functions.)
13. Infections such as late-stage syphilis.

Antibiotics can effectively treat syphilis at any stage, but they cannot reverse the brain damage already done.

"Sometimes dementia runs in families and is inherited. Doctors often suspect an inherited cause if someone younger than fifty has symptoms of dementia."

"Jennifer Thomas raised her hand to speak "It is my understanding the advancement of dementia depends upon what is causing it and the part of the brain that is affected. Dementia may progress slowly over a period of years or quite rapidly. Some patients with dementia do not realize they have mental deterioration. They won't admit their condition and may blame others for their problems. Those who are aware of what is happening may become discouraged and depressed."

"That is my understanding as well," Emma replied. "Also, with certain types of dementia a person's behavior may get out of control. They may become childish in their behavior, angry, and overly dependent. Some become mean and combative."

"There is another condition" added Jane Ruth "called wandering where the person goes for walk from where they are living and becomes lost. This makes it more and more difficult for the family to care for the patient at home."

"Yes, I am very familiar with that" said Emma. "My uncle and aunt had her mother live with them. She had some sort of dementia and after a while began to wander. They had to install locks high up on doors to prevent her from leaving the house alone. People with dementia tend to have a shorter lifespan than the average person their age. This may be due to other conditions such as diabetes or heart disease. I have read that death usually occurs due to lung or kidney infections caused by being bedridden."

"I have a DVD from Terra Nova Films that fits in appropriately here. The name is **Live Outside the Stigma: Confronting the Myths and Stigmas of Alzheimer's disease and other Related Dementia from the Inside Out**. It was produced by Brilliant Image Productions."

Marcie got up and closed the shades to darken the room. Emma continued: "This is the true story of a doctor, Richard Taylor, who was told he had dementia by his neurologist."

The video began with Dr. Taylor dismissing many of the myths and stigmas associated with dementia. Sharing what he had experienced and learned from others in various stages of dementia, he spoke on what it is like to live with dementia, and how others can adjust their thinking and actions to help those diagnosed with the disease to *continue* to live productively. He wrote a book that he referred to as an "insider's manual" on understanding, dealing with, and breaking out of the boundaries of a dementia diagnosis, information he wished he had known early on. His hope is his hindsight will help those newly diagnosed with dementia, as well as caregivers and family members, to get a better understanding of how to live with and/or provide care to persons with dementia."

Several in the class spoke up simultaneously. "How can we get a copy of this 'Insider's Manual'?"

"I think the best way would be to contact Terra Nova Films. I'll get you the phone number," Emma replied.

Emma looked at her watch. "This has been a lively discussion. I have enjoyed it and hope you did as well. Next week we will discuss Alzheimer's disease and animal and music therapy. Have a good week, all."

The class applauded as they rose to leave. "Good lesson, Emma," said Dale from Group Eight.

THE SUNSET YEARS

Emma smiled. "Thank you, thank you very much."

Dr. Arthur walked up to Emma. "Would you walk with me to the cafeteria and have a cup of coffee? I have an idea I would like to discuss with you."

"I'd love to," she replied with a smile.

The hospital cafeteria offered a wide variety of food for its patrons including a large salad buffet, hot meal selection, custom made sandwiches and hamburgers, along with a selection of tempting desserts. The dining room was a large open area with seating for at least one hundred diners. One wall had been built with floor to ceiling windows providing a view to those inside of a well-landscaped courtyard complete with an array of colorful flowers, mature trees and shrubs. The backdrop of rocks and boulders complimented the multilevel flagstone base giving the area a feeling of being semi-enclosed. Some visitors thought of it as a peaceful grotto, a place for privacy and quiet. Sitting outside one could hear the gentle rippling of water as it followed the path of the man-made stream. A number of tables and chairs had been strategically placed and several people were eating, visiting, and just enjoying the surroundings.

After picking up their coffee Emma and Dr. Arthur decided to join the folks outside. Finding a table they sat down and chatted awhile about the class and the topic of discussion for today – dementia. Applauding Emma on her presentation of the subject, Dr. Arthur then stated the real reason he wanted to speak with her. "I was wondering if I could do the presentation on Alzheimer's disease next week. It's personal with me. As you know, my mother has Alzheimer's. It is a dreadful disease and I have done a bit of research on the subject."

"That would be fantastic," Emma responded. "It would be an honor to have you present and the class would enjoy hearing from one of their own."

"I'm sorry about your mom. It must pain you when you go

to visit her and she doesn't recognize you, realize you are her son."

"There are times when she does know me, but many times she doesn't and, yes, it is distressful."

They continued to visit awhile until their coffee was finished. Then John said, "Thank you. I've enjoyed visiting with you. I've got to get back to work."

"And I need to go home" Emma replied. "Have a good day."

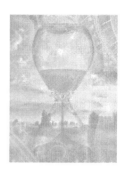

Thus aged men, full loth and slow,
The vanities of life forego,
And count their youthful follies o'er
'Til memory lends her light no more."

Sir Walter Scott

Chapter Five
Alzheimer's disease

The week had gone by quickly. Emma and Jon had taken a long weekend in the mountains. It was over too soon. She was eagerly anticipating class today and Dr. Arthur's presentation. The students arrived and quickly everyone was seated. Emma, standing at the front of the class revealed, "Today, Dr. Arthur will lead the discussion on Alzheimer's disease."

Dr. Arthur stood up and walked to the front of the room. "Thank you, Emma."

"Alzheimer's disease is personal for me. As many of you

know my mother has the Alzheimer's disease and I know only too well what it is and the damage it does. The nerve cells of the brain gradual deteriorate and as these cells die loss of memory occurs, and thinking and language skills are slowly lost. Alzheimer's is not a normal part of aging, but age is the most common cause of dementia in those over 65. Does anyone know who discovered the disease?"

Dr. Jennifer Thomas stood up and answered, "I don't know exactly but I believe it was a German doctor."

"You are right," replied Dr. Arthur. "The origin of the disease dates back to 1906 when a German doctor, Alois Alzheimer, presented the story of a 51 year old woman who suffered from a rare brain disorder. Upon her death an autopsy showed plaque and tangles in her brain, which today are the characteristics of Alzheimer's."

"Does anyone know the warning signs of Alzheimer's?"

Claire Donahue in Group Five stood up. "My aunt who had Alzheimer's lived with our family. She passed away a few years ago. I remember at first she had difficulty remembering what she did yesterday, or what she had for breakfast. Then as the disease progressed her personality changed. One day she said to me: '*Claire, what do those numbers mean?*' I looked at her and she pointed to the clock. She didn't know what it was. The last thing I remember was she had received a letter from her sister and although she could read it, she didn't understand the words she had read."

Dr. Arthur looked at her and said, "I'm so sorry, Claire. Alzheimer's is truly a debilitating disease and hard on the whole family."

"It was hard on all of us, especially my mother," Claire responded.

Dr. Arthur continued: "Experts in the field have

identified common warning signs of the disease. These symptoms slowly get worse and become more permanent." He walked over to the large paper chart and flipped over the top page. "I have listed the symptoms here."

1. Unable to remember recent events, names.
2. Mixed up, confused about time and place.
3. Difficulty doing everyday tasks, such as brushing teeth or combing hair.
4. Difficulty speaking in complete sentences, having conversations, and following directions.
5. Loss of decision making ability; poor judgment.
6. Irritability, withdrawing from others.
7. Inability to do complex mental assignments such as settling their checkbook.
8. Having visions of things not there.

"When examining a patient, there are two basic symptoms doctors look for. It is important to identify them correctly because the treatment used depends on the symptoms present. The first type is loss of intellectual ability. That includes loss of memory, in particular, short term memory; the inability to communicate, to write and/or speak; the inability to do daily living activities such as brushing teeth and getting dressed; inability to interpret bodily signals, such as needing use the bathroom, or pain in the body."

"The second class of symptoms is of a psychiatric nature. These symptoms include hallucinations, personality changes, depression, and delusions. Patients with psychiatric symptoms tend to have more behavioral issues than those patients with the cognitive or intellectual disorders."

"Of these symptoms listed on the chart, which would be cognitive and which psychiatric?" he asked the class. Dr. Parsons raised his hand.

"Yes, Dr. Parsons."

"I would say they are all cognitive with the exception of numbers 6 and 8."

"I believe you're right" replied Dr. Arthur. He smiled at Dr. Parsons.

Continuing, he said, "Most people are not aware that there are two types of Alzheimer's disease. The first, familial Alzheimer's disease, (FAD) also known as Early Onset Alzheimer's, is passed directly by a mutated gene from one generation to another. This form of the disease is usually seen in middle-aged people that are between the ages of 30 and 60. The other, sporadic Alzheimer's disease is more prevalent. This disease is not inherited, but people developing this disease may have a disposition in their genetic makeup that may make them more susceptible to the illness. These patients are usually between the ages of sixty and seventy years of age, defined by some as the onset of being elderly" he stated and smiled.

"Does anyone know how Alzheimer's is diagnosed by doctors?"

"I'll give it a crack," said Dr. Parsons as he smiled and stood up once again. It was obvious the two men were friends. "I believe the first thing they would do is to take a complete medical history of the patient followed by a physical examination. Then they would conduct tests such as brain scans and neuro-psychological tests that measure memory, attention, language skills, and problem solving abilities."

"Very good, Dr. Parsons. You do know your stuff." John grinned and the class, as well as Dr. Parsons, laughed at Dr. Arthur's comment. Arthur continued: "Diagnoses can be up to 90 percent correct, but can only be confirmed by an autopsy. Proper diagnosis is critical because there are other causes of memory problems which can be treated."

THE SUNSET YEARS

Dr. Arthur walked over to the chart. "I have listed the seven stages of Alzheimer's disease here. These stages were developed by Dr. Barry Reisberg, the clinical director of the New York University School of Medicine's Silberstein Aging and Dementia Research Center. Not all patients have the same symptoms and some of the stages may overlap with each other."

Stage 1: No impairment
Stage 2: Very mild decline
Stage 3: Mild decline
Stage 4: Moderate decline
Stage 5: Moderately severe decline
Stage 6: Severe decline
Stage 7: Very severe decline

"In the first stage there are no memory problems and no symptoms of dementia."

"In the second stage there may be a slight decline in intellectual abilities. There may be memory lapses, but no symptoms of dementia."

"In stage three memory and concentration problems appear and are recognizable by some friends, family members, and/or colleagues. They may have trouble remembering a name when they are introduced to someone new. They may not remember what they have just read, and may have difficulty planning for an event or occasion."

"In Stage Four, still in the early stages of the disease, the patient may forget recent events and may not be able to do simple arithmetic. Complex tasks such as paying bills or having guests over for dinner and planning for the meal becomes a challenge. They may forget their own history, and may become moody or withdrawn."

"Stage Five begins the mid-stage of the disease. During this period the patient may not remember his own address or telephone number or where they went to high school or college. They may not know what day it is or what to wear appropriate for weather conditions. They still are able to eat on their own and use the bathroom by themselves."

"By stage six there is severe loss of intellectual ability. They memory issues continue to get worse, personality changes may occur, and the patient needs help with his daily activities. They may not know where they are and may not remember the names of family members or their caregiver. They have trouble controlling their bladder or bowels. At this stage they may begin to wander."

"Stage seven, the final phase of the disease, patients lose their ability to respond to their surroundings, to have a conversation, and eventually control their movements. They may still be able to say words and phrases. They need help with their daily activities including eating or using the bathroom. Some lose the ability to smile, sit without support, or hold their heads up. Reflexes become abnormal, muscles become inflexible, and the ability to swallow is compromised. It is very disheartening to watch someone you love slowly decline."

"What is the prognosis?" asked Susan. "I have read the disease can progress from two to twenty years."

"On the average" Dr. Arthur replied, "individuals live from eight to ten years from diagnosis. Most develop co-existing illnesses and many die from pneumonia. Alzheimer's disease is among the top 10 leading causes of death in the U.S."

"Is anyone familiar with the statistics on Alzheimer's?" No one volunteered. John walked over to the large chart and flipped over the top page. There he had listed some of the current statistics.

- Early onset Alzheimer's and some form of dementia is said to occur in a half million Americans younger than age 65.
- As many as 5.1 million Americans may have the disease

and with the aging population, the frequency of the disease is likely to grow. The risk of developing the illness rises with advanced age.

- About 25 percent of those with the disease are cared for by their families.
- Current research from the National Institute on Aging indicates that the occurrence of Alzheimer's disease doubles every five years beyond age sixty-five.
- According to the U.S. Census Bureau the numbers of people age sixty-five and older will more than double between 2010 and 2050 to 20 percent of the population; likewise, those eighty-five and older will rise three-fold, to 19 million.

Dr. Arthur continued. "The cost to the nation of caring for people with Alzheimer's is staggering, estimated at $100 billion dollars a year. Businesses alone in the United States figure their cost is more than $60 billion. Those costs are determined by absenteeism, insurance costs, and lost productivity."

"Does anyone know what it costs annually to care for one individual with Alzheimer's?"

"Expensive" Dr. Sparks answered.

"Yes it is. About $30,000, but I have read the actual cost depends on the stage of the disease and it can range from $18,000 to $36,000. Personally, I believe that might be low especially if the patient is in a specialized nursing home facility."

Continuing, he said, "There is some research being done on the disease. No one knows what causes it, but the greatest risk factor is age. Some think it may be caused by many factors including genetic makeup, serious head injuries, overproduction of toxic free radicals, and oxidative damage to neurons."

"What are free radicals?" asked Lucy Rose. "I've heard that term a lot, but really never understood what they were."

"Free radicals, also known as radicals, are carbon-based particles or molecules responsible for aging, tissue damage, and possibly some diseases. They are very unstable, and look to bond with other molecules. Antioxidants, present in many foods, prevent free radicals from harming healthy tissue."

"And what does 'oxidative damage' mean?" she asked.

Looking at Lucy he thought: *I'm impressed. She is not intimidated to ask questions.* Answering her he said "Oxidative damage is caused by free radicals that have not been neutralized by antioxidants and cause physical stress on the body, which is why *what we eat* is so important." He emphasized 'what we eat'. "A physical example of oxidative damage with which we are all familiar is rust on metal."

"Does anyone know of any preventative measures people can do to ward off the risk of Alzheimer's disease?" Sarah Driscoll asked.

Dr. Arthur walked over to the chart and flipped over the top page. "The following I found on the Alzheimer's Prevention website. It stated: '*brain health begins in the womb and needs to be promoted across your lifespan.*' It listed things people can do to promote brain health. I have not included everything. For more information go to their website: http://www.alzprevention.org/index.php."

- Nutrition: Do not overeat. Eat healthy foods. Increase your intake of Omega 3 fatty acids, walnuts and unsalted nuts.
- Eat more foods that contain antioxidants, i.e.

vitamins, minerals, and other nutrients that protect and repair cells from damage caused by free radicals. These would include colorful fruits and vegetables such as grapes, apples, cantaloupe, berries, and leafy green vegetables. The USDA recommends five servings of fruit and vegetables a day.

- Decrease eating processed foods and red meats.
- Eat one 'sit down' meal a day with others.
- Socialization: As we get older we should not isolate ourselves from others, but maintain and build friendships including family members.
- Develop hobbies. Do not retire from life.
- Physical Activity: Walk daily. Tending a garden, aerobic exercises, even dancing, are all good physical activities.
- Mental Stimulation: Do anything that will stimulate your brain such as learn a second language, learn a musical instrument, play board games, travel, listen to music, and more.
- Spirituality: Learn to meditate. Learn relaxation procedures. Attend a place of worship.

"Does anyone have any questions?"

"What harm does eating red meat do to the body and brain?" asked Lucy.

"Red meat contain large quantities of iron, and it is thought that iron build-up can cause oxidative damage to brain cells as well as disruption of nerve signals."

"Have you ever heard of 'Sun downing'?" asked Marcie.

"Yes. Sun downing or Sundowners Syndrome is an emotional episode that occurs in patients with some forms of dementia, but more often with Alzheimer's disease. It is a type of behavior that usually happens as the sun begins to go down and shadows appear. These patients may become very stressed, anxious and unsettled, develop mood swings, or become baffled and irritated with their own confusion. Some experience agitation while trying to sleep, and then begin pacing or wandering. Others get upset with their caregiver and start yelling at him or her."

"What can be done to help these patients?" asked Susan.

"It is thought that having a regular sleeping schedule and daily routine can reduce the anxiety and confusion. Not allowing afternoon naps, but taking the patient on walks during the day helps to encourage sleep at night. Also no coffee, hot chocolate, or any drinks with caffeine except in the mornings."

"Are there any more questions?"

"Have you ever read anything about the relationship between Alzheimer's disease and diabetes?" asked Marion Mahoney.

"Yes. Some researchers believe that Alzheimer's disease is now linked more closely with diabetes and can be controlled by diet. Some have named it Type 3 Diabetes or Diabetes of the Brain. As you well know, insulin regulates blood sugar in the body, but as people eat lots of food that are filled with fat and sugar, eventually the cells become overwhelmed and insulin resistant. The excess sugar causes inflammation and/or infection in the body and eventually diseases of the heart, nerves, and even eyes. When it reaches the brain, memory is impaired and according to some, Alzheimer's disease develops. There is much, much more information on the Internet with regards to Alzheimer's and diet."

"What are nitrosamines?" asked Jim Howard.

"I'm glad I prepared for this class" said Dr. Arthur, smiling. You have asked me some tough questions. Nitrosamines are formed when sodium nitrites, added to food as preservatives to prevent salmonella infection, combine with stomach acid to form a chemical agent known as nitrosamine. Many *processed* foods such as cheese, hotdogs, smoked meats (bacon, turkey, ham) even beer are contaminated with nitrosamines. Also, when foods are prepared at high temperatures by frying or flame broiling, nitrates and nitrites are changed into nitrosamines. There have been some laboratory experiments that have confirmed even limited exposure to nitrosamines can cause Alzheimer's type brain degeneration, dementia, diabetes, fatty liver disease and obesity. It may even be the root cause to those diseases. To protect yourself check labels carefully and avoid foods that contain sodium nitrites. Avoid processed foods, and choose to eat organic products."

"Is there any treatment for Alzheimer's disease" asked Lucy.

"Research is being done on various drugs continually to alleviate symptoms and/or to slow or reverse behavioral issues, as well as to halt the disease itself. But, as of today there is no cure, no magic pill. Thank you for asking, Lucy."

"One more question" asked Jennifer Thomas. Is there any link that you know of between Alzheimer's and Aluminum?"

"There has been some research on that, but I am not familiar with it."

Looking at Emma, Dr. Arthur said, "Thank you for allowing me to give this presentation." He walked to his group and sat down. As he did the class applauded loudly.

"Good job," they responded as he sat down.

"*Thank you*, Dr. Arthur. You gave an extremely informative presentation and I feel certain we all learned a great deal about Alzheimer's disease. Let's take a short break and when we return we will discuss animal and music therapy. We have Dr. Chu from the University of Nebraska here to speak on the value of music therapy."

LAUREL HALL

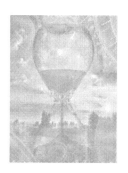

There is in souls a sympathy with sounds,
And as the mind is pitch'd, the ear is pleas'd
With melting airs of martial, brisk or grave,
Some chord in unison with what we hear
Is touch'd within us, and the heart replies.
W. Cowper

Chapter Six
Animal and Music Therapy

Within fifteen minutes the class was seated. Emma proceeded to the front of the room and began to speak. "There are a number of different therapies used in working with patients having Alzheimer's disease and dementia. These include occupational therapy, light therapy, art therapy, massage therapy and others, and each claims different benefits. You can read about the various therapies on the

Internet. Not all therapies work with every patient and not all patients are suited for the different types of therapy. Today we will concentrate on two: animal therapy and music therapy."

"As dementia and Alzheimer's disease advance, patients are more and more at risk of isolation and loneliness. Having a pet come into their life can be a blessing. Dogs give unconditional love and perhaps, that is why when people think of animal therapy, dogs come to mind. However, cats, rabbits, birds, fish, and even horses can be used as therapy animals."

"Who can give me a benefit of bringing a dog to visit Alzheimer or dementia patients?"

Emma saw a hand go up. "Yes, Dr. Evans."

"People with dementia often lack the physical touch we all crave; a dog can provide that".

"That's right. Who can give me another benefit? Yes, Marion."

"Allowing the patient to pet and love on the dog can be emotionally rewarding, providing emotional stimulation, entertainment, and maybe even the recollection of fond memories of previous pets".

"Very good." Who can provide another? Yes, Muriel."

"They can provide a glimmer of happiness, especially if their surroundings are very depressing."

"That's so true, Muriel. Any others? Yes, Dr. Parsons."

"A visit from a loving dog or cat can help relieve loneliness and depression, as well as lessen aggressive or hyperactive behavior. It also provides a means for positive nonverbal communication."

"Thank you. All good reasons. How about fish? What can they do?" Walter Carbonera raised his hand. "Yes, Walter."

"A beautiful, well decorated aquarium can be mesmerizing, watching the colorful fish sway in and out of the rocks, plants, and other artifacts in the water."

THE SUNSET YEARS

"That's true, Walter.   In some studies nursing homes which had fish tanks stocked with brilliantly colored fish have helped to inhibit disorderly behavior and improve eating habits of some patients. The combination of color and sound offers an inspiring experience, and watching the fish move around in various patterns keeps the patient interested.   In another study patients appeared to be more relaxed and alert when around the fish.   What about horses? They seem so big to take to a nursing home." Emma asked and smiled.

Dr. Arthur stood. "I read about a study in Ohio where some patients in the early stages of Alzheimer's have had the opportunity to work with horses, learning how to clean, brush, and care for horse, as well as how to put a halter on the animal and walk it. They enjoy taking pictures of the horses and just being around them."

"So the patients actually go to a horse farm or some facility that has horses?"

"Yes" he replied, rather amused. "As a general rule horses do not go to nursing homes."

"I have a friend who, for a number of years, had two large tropical birds," said Emma. "By large, I mean ten to twelve inches tall. I don't recall the types of birds, but their names were Brutus and Caesar. Caesar was a beautiful white bird with a yellow crown on his head; Brutus, a large blue and gold colored bird.   They were well-behaved and very well-trained.   Kelly would take them to nursing homes on a monthly basis for the residents to enjoy. Brutus would sit on his perch and watch everyone, while Caesar would walk around visiting the patients, feeling right at home. Watching the residents enjoy the birds, petting them, and seeing firsthand the pleasure it gave them, made going to the home a joy for Kelly. The birds seemed to enjoy the outing as well."

"Music is another form of therapy which can have a positive effect on people. Today we have Dr. Chu from the University of Nebraska to speak to us on music therapy. Please give him a warm welcome. Dr. Chu." As the class applauded, Emma took a seat in the back of the room.

"It is a distinct pleasure for me to be here today and share with you the current information on the use of music with patients having dementia or Alzheimer's disease. Using music with Alzheimer's patients has been found to reduce anxiety and improve social and behavioral problems. Even in advanced stages it has been found patients can tap to the music or sing songs they knew in childhood. Some studies suggest that general information and memory of music remains preserved in the brain even though reasoning, learning, attention, and memory abilities are impaired. Music provides a way for patients to connect even after speaking has become challenging."

"It has been known for years that music has a calming effect on people and helps diffuse stress and tension. With the deterioration of the brain, the body's functions fail as well. All five senses are affected, but with patients who have this disease, the sense of hearing is usually the first to go. As long as the patient can still hear, music therapy will most likely be beneficial."

"The Alzheimer's Association is familiar with the value of music therapy. Listening to music they knew in their youth can stir long-term memories in an elderly person. At the same time looking at photographs while listening to music can stimulate other memories as well."

Dr. Mahoney raised her hand. "How and why does it work?"

Dr. Chu responded, "Music is presumed to be beneficial because it reduces stress by modifying how patients identify sound. It can help patients understand their environment, and may decrease any fear or anxiety they may have. Music can also provide a method for patients to communicate and interact with others."

"Thank you."

Dr. Chu continued. "One study with Alzheimer's patients showed how music affected secretion levels of the brain chemical melatonin, a hormone linked with various mood behaviors such as depression and aggression. It also helped the patient sleep better. The good news here was higher levels of this hormone continued for weeks after music therapy had ended."

"In another study it was found that patients showed significant improvement in speaking with others. In yet another study some patients showed improvement in their reasoning abilities, social skills and behavior. Music therapy will not cure Alzheimer's disease or dementia, but the use of music seems to have positive results on the symptoms of the disease and can lead to an improved quality of life for both the patient and his or her caregiver."

"Emma obtained a video for you to watch from Terra Nova Films, *Beyond the Music:* **the Power of Music with People who are Living with Dementia and Other Age- related Conditions.** It was produced by Sally Jane Archer and Alkeiya Brown, a musical therapist. I have previewed it and think it is excellent. This film shows actual footage of how music therapy stimulates memory and social interactions while reducing behavioral, cognitive, and emotional problems."

Dr. Chu started the video. It acknowledged the power of music to surpass the challenges of dementia, and showed actual non-responsive, non-verbal residents suddenly smiling, singing, moving, and interacting with others when engaged through music. Dr. Chu stopped the video and said: "These before-and-after glimpses of residents 'reconnecting' encourage us to believe that the use of music therapy as a method to boost quality of life for residents is genuine."

Restarting the DVD, the video narrator discussed the capability of the brain to modify its own organization and purpose through thought and activity and the soothing effect of music. As the video ended Dr. Chu said, "This DVD was based on the work of the registered music therapist I mentioned earlier, Alkeiya Brown. She has had widespread experience working with all ages from the very young to very old in the field of music therapy."

Marcie stood up to ask a question. "As a lay person with a family member or friend with dementia or Alzheimer's, how does one go about using music with the patient?"

Dr. Chu looked at her and spoke. "Again, it all depends on the stage of the disease. In general, I would try some of the following:

- Find music the person liked when they were younger. Download music on your iPhone or a CD. Pandora is a good source for music. Create a playlist of songs they liked and play the songs while you are visiting.
- If the patient is in the early to middle stages use a karaoke player for the patient to sing along with the music.
- Make listening to music a fun experience. Use clapping or toe tapping to enhance the involvement.
- Bring photographs to look at together while the music is playing.
- Use music to create the mood you want. If the person is agitated use a calming piece of music to create a calm environment. To boost spirits use happy songs from the person's past.

THE SUNSET YEARS

- Get rid of competing noises. Close windows, doors, and turn off the TV. Don't make the music too loud."

"In closing, music has always been enjoyable and relaxing to people. Doctors are just beginning to understand how music affects the heart and mind. With music the victim is given a chance to reconnect with past memories and with the world around them. It gives them an opportunity to hold onto something that makes them feel whole again, even if for a short time."

"Thank you so very much, Dr. Chu for coming to Colorado and sharing your knowledge on music therapy with us." The class gave a big round of applause.

"Thank you for having me. It has been my pleasure."

"Next week we will have a guest speaker to tell us about federal and state laws with regards to elder abuse," Emma said. She picked up the bowl with the group numbers and pulled out one piece of paper. "Group Two, you will present on Physical Abuse. Have a good week, all."

As the class rose, many students walked over to Dr. Chu to ask questions of him. They had clearly been impressed with the thought-provoking information he had shared.

LAUREL HALL

"Law does not the least restraint
upon our freedom. But maintain' t;
Or if it does, it's for our good,
To give us freer latitude;
For wholesome law preserve us free,
By stinting of our liberty."
Samuel Butler

Chapter Seven
Federal and State Laws

I t was a beautiful morning. The temperature was in the low seventies with partly cloudy skies. The forecast had said it might rain. *Slim chance*, thought Emma, *but we really do need the rain.* Every time rain was predicted it rarely came. Walking into the air-conditioned building felt wonderful. Taking the elevator to the sixth floor she found some students already there. They seemed eager and looking forward to class. After ten minutes or so the class was seated. Standing by the door Emma said, "Today we have a guest speaker who will speak to us on federal and state laws regarding elder abuse. Please welcome Attorney Peter Crowell."

Crowell walked to the front of the class where a large paper chart had been placed while Emma took a seat in the back of the room. On the first page he had written: "Federal Laws". Beneath that was written "Elder Justice Act (EJA)".

Turning to the class he said "Listening to someone speak on the law is like listening to a lecture in history class. It can be boring." The class laughed. "I will do my best to not be dull, but no promises."

"Both federal and state laws address elder abuse, neglect and exploitation, but state law is the primary source for penalties, remedies and protections. A few federal laws speak explicitly to elder abuse and neglect, but none of these laws provide comprehensive procedures for state or local programs. It is the states that provide support services for victims of elder abuse."

"Does anyone know when the first act was created to deal with senior citizens?" No one raised their hand. "Aha." Then he said, not in a mean way, "Why am I not surprised?"

"The first act to deal with senior citizens was the Older Americans Act (OAA) passed by Congress in 1965 as an answer to concerns about a lack of community services for older people. The initial legislation gave the government the right to provide monies in the form of grants to the states for community planning and social services, research and development, as well as personnel training in the field of aging. The OAA developed the definitions of elder abuse, It established the Administration on Aging (AoA) to administer grant programs and serve as the Federal focal point on matters concerning older people. Today, the OAA is thought to be the major channel for the organization and delivery of social and nutrition services to older people and their caregivers. It was amended in 2006 under Title VII."

"Has anyone heard of the EJA?" No one volunteered. Peter laughed. "I guess law is not your top priority."

Crowell continued. "The Elder Justice Act was introduced into legislation in 2002 and enacted into law in March, 2010 as part of the Patient Protection and Affordable Care Act, sometimes called 'Obamacare'." Peter smiled and continued. "It was the first piece of federal legislation passed to provide a specific source of government monies to address elder abuse, neglect and exploitation. This Act coordinates federal elder abuse programs within the Office of the Secretary of Health and Human Services and establishes an Elder Abuse Coordinating Council with members having skill in elder abuse prevention, exposure, treatment, mediation or prosecution. This council is comprised of the HHS secretary, Attorney General, federal department and agency heads and 27 members of the public with expertise in elder abuse, prevention, detection, treatment, intervention, and/or prosecution. To date, however, Congress has appropriated no money for implementation of the Elder Justice Act."

"Who can tell me they don't the difference between 'authorize' and 'appropriate' with regards to Congress and passing bills?"

Sharon Linn raised her hand. "I believe when Congress authorizes a piece of legislation, that means it passes and become a law. But, if Congress does not appropriate money for it, the bill doesn't get funded and what it can do is very limited."

"Absolutely right," said Peter Crowell. "When the OAA was enacted in 1965 it was funded by Congress and for many years. This year, 2013, it's a different story. Some members of Congress do not want to fund the Affordable Care Act and as a result, these programs are in jeopardy."

"When (and if) the EJA is fully funded it will provide some of the following," he said, and pointed to the chart.

- Forensic Centers
- Long-term care staff
- Adult Protective Services
- Elder Abuse Investigation
- Responsibilities of owners of long-term care

"Does anyone know what a 'forensic center' is or what it does?"

Dr. Howard from the back of the room spoke up. "I would suppose it has something to do with the law."

"Right," said Crowell. "There will be four stationary and six mobile forensic centers. Their purpose is to develop legal gauges, procedures for legal involvement, legal know-how, and ability to collect legal proof of elder abuse."

"The next item, long-term care staff, includes employing, teaching and retaining staff, as well as programs to improve management practices and the adoption of requirements for the electronic exchange of medical data."

"Is anyone familiar with the APS?" the attorney asked.

Dr. Webber raised his hand. "I believe it has something to do with protecting people from abuse."

"It does. Adult Protective Services (APS) was created in each state to look into reports on suspected abuse, neglect and financial exploitation of the elderly. Government funds issued by the OAA helped to provide monies to the states for these programs."

"The fourth bullet refers to a national institute for training, technical assistance and the development of best practices which was created by the EJA to improve the reporting of elder abuse in long-term care facilities."

"And finally, owners, operators and employees of long-term care facilities must report suspected crimes committed in their facilities to the Health and Human Services Secretary (HHS). They must also provide 60 days' notice in writing to the HHS Secretary and to the state of a facility's impending closure. The notice must include a strategy for transfer and satisfactory relocation of all residents."

"Another provision of the Patient Protection and Affordable Care Act requires the HHS Secretary to establish a nationwide program for national and state background checks on prospective employees who will have direct access to patients in long-term care facilities. This is very important for the protection of the residents."

Crowell flipped the top sheet of the paper chart over. On the top he had written "Administration on Aging." Beneath was listed:

- National Center on Elder Abuse (NCEA)
- Violence against Women Act
- Elder Abuse Victim Act

"The National Center on Elder Abuse is a program of the Administration on Aging. The NCEA along with other organizations promotes and supports elder abuse awareness ideas, gathers responses to abuse by experts in various disciplines, along with professional training and education for personnel in the field."

"The next bullet, Violence against Women Act, established federal domestic violence crimes that may be applied in cases of elder abuse. It includes committing or attempting to commit a crime of violence against an intimate partner, by following or bothering in any way, (in person, by mail or computer), as well as the violation of a qualifying protection order".

"The Elder Abuse Victims Act of 2009, which is still pending in the Senate Judiciary Committee, approves federal contributions for training state and local attorneys, courts, and law enforcement personnel conduct in elder justice-related matters. It establishes the Elder Serve Victim grant program to assist and manage emergency services to victims of elder abuse."

"Well, that is a basic overview of federal laws with regards to elder abuse. There is much, much more, too much to accomplish in this setting, but until the Affordable Care Act is funded, the EJA can do only a limited amount."

"Are there any questions?"

"How does the average person find out about all these provisions for the elderly?" asked Hai Wong.

"Both federal and state governments are trying to make people aware of these provisions. For example, in Colorado a booklet called *ANSWERS ON AGING* is provided by Larimer County, Office on Aging. It is an excellent resource guide for information on housing, caregiver support, transportation services, in-home care, and much more. Trouble is most people don't read these kinds of magazine because they feel they are not applicable to them at this time. Each of us needs to be knowledgeable of what is available, so if someone else needs help, perhaps we can guide them in the right direction. The programs on the federal level each have a website that discusses their part with regards to elder abuse, neglect, and exploitation."

"States address elder abuse in numerous legal areas, including Adult Protective Service laws, criminal codes, probate, trusts and estate codes, family law, and civil remedies. Legal systems vary widely and in most states the laws related to elder abuse may be found in several code sections. I have written the major categories of state laws addressing elder abuse below" he said pointing to the chart.

- Services to victims
- Long-Term Care residents
- Laws applicable to elder abuse
- Domestic abuse
- Financial exploitation

"All states have Adult Protective Services (APS) or Elder Protective Services (EPS) laws that approve and control the providing of services in cases of elder abuse. Some states have both EPS and APS statutes, and some states have more than one APS law. These laws set up systems for reporting and looking into suspected elder abuse and for providing care to victims."

"All states also have laws establishing a Long-Term Care Ombudsman Program. These programs advocate for the rights, safety and other interests of long-term care facility residents. Approximately 15 states also have separate laws that address abuse, neglect and exploitation of these residents."

"All states have general criminal laws on offenses that can be applied in cases of elder abuse. A few states provide increased penalties for abusing older adults, while some states specify elder abuse as one or more separate crimes."

"Several states recently have taken aim at the financial exploitation of older persons. For example, Maryland passed a law requiring monetary institutions to report suspected financial abuse of older persons to APS or law enforcement within 24 hours of the suspicious activity. Missouri amended its elder abuse law to include undue influence as an act that, when committed against an elderly or disabled person, constitutes the crime of financial exploitation."

"All states provide civil remedies for domestic abuse violence including criminal statutes and civil protection orders. Examples of other legal remedies include liability for identity theft, financial exploitation, or misleading practices and removal of durable power of attorney".

"Most states have laws designed to protect the safety and financial interests of the elderly, disabled or vulnerable adults. All states provide protections of adults with some impairment of capacity through guardianship of the person, financial matters and/or property".

"State laws vary and what is true in one state may not be true in another. A wealth of information is available on the Internet if you are interested in learning more."

"Let's talk about our state, Colorado. Unfortunately, according to the American Bar Association's Commission on Law and Aging, Colorado remains one of four states that do not require anyone, be it doctor, social worker, or others, to report elder abuse to the police or the APS. However, there is a possibility that there will be new legislation soon."

"Have you ever heard of the elderly man pushing for mandatory reporting laws for elder abuse?" asked Attorney Dobson from Group Eight.

"Yes," Peter replied. "I was reading in the Denver newspaper about a gentleman, now in his eighties, who has been working for years to get a law passed in Colorado making reporting of elderly abuse by professionals mandatory."

"What are the other states that do not require mandatory reporting?" asked Marcie from Group Two.

"I believe they are New York, and North and South Dakota. Anymore questions?"

"What does Ombudsman mean?" asked Lucy.

"It's like a watchdog program, a supervisory panel to overlook state programs."

"Thank you," she replied.

"Are there any other questions?" There being none, Emma walked to the front of the class and thanked Counselor Crowell for his presentation. "Let's give a round of applause for Mr. Crowell?" The class stood and gave him a standing ovation.

"Let's take a short break after which Group Two will present on physical abuse."

A few of the students stood back to visit with the attorney asking him further questions. Emma was pleased that Peter Crowell had done such an outstanding job with his presentation.

LAUREL HALL

THE SUNSET YEARS

"...Pain clings cruelly to us,
Like the gnawing sloth on the
Deer's tender haunches... *
Keats

Chapter Eight
Physical Abuse

While the students were milling about the refreshment table, Emma opened her briefcase, and pulled out a banner, which she then taped to the wall. On it was printed in bold letters: **"ELDER ABUSE IS A VIOLATION OF HUMAN RIGHTS, A SIGNIFICANT CAUSE OF ILLNESS, INJURY, AND A SIGNIFICANT LOSS OF PRODUCTIVITY, ISOLATION AND DESPAIR".** That was a statement the World Health Organization had made in 2002.

Soon the students were reseated. Emma began the class. "Today, Group Two will give their presentation on physical abuse. Group Two, the floor is yours," she said smiling as she walked to the back of the room.

Group Two walked to the front of the class. Dr. Arthur spoke first. "We obtained much of our information from The National Committee for the Prevention of Elder Abuse (NCPEA). This organization was established in 1988 and serves as the nation's clearinghouse and resource for elder abuse and neglect. In doing my research I read that a person age sixty or above is considered elderly, and eighty or over is considered 'old elderly.' Personally, I feel that needs to be redefined. I believe it should be more like senior citizen begins at sixty-five, elderly at eighty, and old elderly at ninety and above." John l a u g h e d, as did the class. "After all, I don't like the idea of being called 'elderly' next year."

Emma smiled and then began laughing with the others. "I agree with those definitions," she said.

Next, Dr. Arthur introduced his co-worker and teammate. "Let me introduce you to Sharon Linn, another member of our group. She also works in my office."

"Thank you, Dr. Arthur. I found a video from Terra Nova Films in Chicago and our group felt it would be appropriate to s h o w at this time. It is called *Just to have a peaceful life.*"

"Would someone darken the room please," asked Emma.

Marcie walked over to the wall of glass and by pushing a button the shades closed automatically.

The class watched the ten-minute video in silence. It portrayed the true story of a woman who was married to a physically abusive husband for 45 years. They had five children who were also physically abused by the husband. She had left him three times when the children were small only to return because of financial problems. She kept hoping he would change as he got older, mellow out, so to speak, but that did not happen. She finally left him; she went to a battered woman's shelter at age 61 only to soon return again because of health problems. She died at age 63 without ever achieving the peaceful life for which she longed.

At the end of the video no one in the room spoke. Marcie opened the curtains and returned to the front of the room. Sharon broke the silence. "That video is a true story and the woman in the video was the real woman, not an actress."

"That makes it so much more personal when you realize she was the actual woman the video portrayed," Emma commented.

Marcie spoke next. "So how do we define elder abuse and elder physical abuse and who are the people that commit these atrocities?" Answering her own question she said, "According to NCPEA, elder abuse is *'any form of mistreatment that results in harm or loss to an older person and is generally divided into categories.'* Physical abuse is one of those categories and is defined as, *'physical force or violence that results in bodily injury, pain, or impairment'*. It includes assault, battery, and inappropriate restraint."

"And who are the offenders?" she asked and then answered. "Believe it or not, it is usually family members - sons, daughters, grandchildren as well as other relatives, and/or acquaintances. These perpetrators are likely to be unmarried, and live with their victims. They are usually unemployed and may have alcohol or substance abuse problems. Some are the caregivers for those they abuse."

Dr. Sparks from Group Three raised his hand. "What is the difference when a spouse is the perpetrator?"

"Good question," Marcie replied. "Physical abuse that is committed by spouses or intimate partners in order to gain power and control over the victim is described as domestic violence."

"Are some seniors more at risk for abuse than others?" asked Dr. Howard from Group Seven.

"Victims of physical abuse do not differ significantly from those who are not abused, but I suspect they might not have had a warm, loving relationship with the families in years past." replied Marcie.

"How do you know an elderly person is being abused?" asked Barbara Edwards from Group One.

"I'll answer that," said Rebecca. "That was my homework assignment," she added smiling. "There are a number of physical signs, but no one indicator can be used as proof of abuse. However, patterns or groups of physical indicators may suggest a problem." She flipped over the first paper on a large chart and there she had listed a number of physical indicators:

- Bodily injuries such as broken bones or dislocated joints.
- Cigarette or hot water burns on the body.
- Scrapes or abrasions on the body that look like rope or strap marks
- Internal injuries which cause pain, bleeding (both internal and external), or difficulty with the normal functioning of organs.

"With regards to bruises," she added, there are many kinds of bruises that are usually *not* accidental. Bruising to both arms may indicate a person has been shaken. Bruises that are multicolored may indicate that these bruises are old and were sustained over a period of time. Bruising of the inner thighs may be an indication of sexual abuse. Bruises that wrap around the body might be an indication of physical restraint."

Gary Friend stepped to the front. "Good job, Rebecca.

THE SUNSET YEARS

There are other signs as well. How a patient behaves around a certain person, perhaps like he is afraid of him, might be an indication of abuse. Mysterious injuries where no one can say how they happened or a history of comparable injuries and/or many trips to the hospital can be signs of abuse. "

"How big a problem is elder abuse?" someone asked from the audience.

"I'll get that," Dr. Arthur offered. "In 1996 the number was estimated to be about half a million people. According to the GAO, today it is estimated that 14% of non-institutionalized older Americans are victims of elder abuse, neglect, or exploitation. Experts, however, believe that for every case of elder abuse reported as many as five cases go unreported. Is anyone familiar with the individual losses associated with elder abuse?" he asked.

No one volunteered to answer the question. "Individual losses associated with elder abuse can be alarming. Among them are included the loss of one's independence, home, savings, health, self-esteem, feeling of self-worth, and safety. Also, comparing older people that have been abused with those that haven't, we find that the life expectancy of the abused group is much shorter."

"Are there any more questions?" he asked. There were none. The room exploded in applause. "Thank you," he said and turned around and thanked each member of the team. "Good job, all." Turning back to the class he said, "We prepared a packet of our presentation for each person."

Emma walked to the front of the room. "What a terrific presentation. Thank you, each one of you. Good job!" Picking up the bowl containing the group numbers, she selected two. "Next week, Group Four will present on Psychological and Emotional abuse followed by Group Three on Financial abuse.

Have a good week."

*...all her friends have dealt
treacherously with her,
They are become her enemies.*
Jeremiah, KJV

Chapter Nine
Psychological/Emotional Abuse

E mma arrived early and went to the cafeteria for coffee. There she saw Marcie and Sharon having breakfast. "May I join you?" she asked.

"Absolutely" both replied in unison. They chatted as they ate, and after a short while left together to go to class.

As they walked into the classroom all the seats were occupied. "Today Group Four will present on Emotional Abuse. Are you ready, Group Four?" Emma asked.

"We are," they responded.

"Then the floor is yours," said Emma as she walked to the back and took a seat. Hai Wong, Dr. Garcia, Dr. Thomas, Susan Bonds, and Lucy Rose walked to the front. Hai began.

"Psychological/Emotional abuse is subtle and the person receiving the abuse may not even know it is happening. Even the people causing the abuse may not know they are abusing another. This type of abuse causes emotional pain to the elder. The family member or other person who is responsible for taking care of the older person may insult, threaten, humiliate, or hound the victim through words or actions. He may ignore the elder or isolate him completely from family members, relatives, or friends. This type of abuse can happen in the elder's home, the caregiver's home, or a facility, such as a nursing home. Emotional abuse can be more harmful than physical abuse because it chisels away at a person's belief in himself or herself."

Hai continued. "There are several kinds of emotional abuse and they harm not just the elderly. Emotional abuse is harmful to anyone of any age."

"We decided to do some play-acting for part of our presentation. Our first scene includes Dr. Garcia who plays an elderly father and Lucy, who plays his daughter." Dr. Garcia sits in a chair, looking pensive while Lucy seems a bit frustrated with her father.

Looking at her father she says: "What's the matter, Dad? You look so down."

"Oh, I was just thinking of your mother and how I miss her."

"Dad, she's been dead over five years. You need to move on, get a life. There are senior centers you can go to, get involved in church. Just sitting around and moping like this is no good for you, and it sure as heck doesn't help me. I feel guilty all the time. I don't know what to do!"

"I just feel so lonely without her. You'll understand someday."

"I miss her too, but life goes on." Lucy stood there with her hands on her hips, frustration lining her face.

Hai interrupts. "Lucy shows no empathy for her dad and no regard for his feelings. Let's see how she might have handled it."

Lucy walks over to her dad. Putting her arm on his shoulder she says, "Dad, you look so down today" and gives him a little hug.

"Oh, I was just thinking of your mother and how I miss her," he explains as his eyes begin to mist.

"Dad, I miss Mom too. It seems like only yesterday she left us. I know you miss her terribly. What can I do to help?"

"Nothing, Lucy. Just having you here has been wonderful."

Hai interrupts. "Lucy has acknowledged her father's feelings and lets him know she understands. Thanks, guys."

"Our next scene shows Dr. Thomas and Susan as elderly sisters living together. They are having a conversation on a purchase Jen had just made."

"Jen, what is that? What on earth did you buy that for? You don't need it. You are always spending your money on rubbish!"

"I thought it was pretty, and I liked it. I was planning to give it to little Emily who lives door."

"You don't have that much money, Jen. You need to be more frugal, make wise choices. You never did make wise choices even when you were younger. Just like the man you married. He was such a jerk. I told you so, but you had to find out for yourself."

"Oh, Susan, why are you always so nasty to me? It seems I can never do anything right."

Hai interrupts. "This is obviously not a healthy relationship. Susan feels superior to Jen, tries to control her spending, and makes her feel bad about decisions she has made. Let's visualize another scenario."

"Jen, what is that you purchased?"

"Oh, nothing. It's just a little figurine."

Susan picks it up and holds it gently. "It's very pretty. I like the colors. Where do you plan to put it?"

"I thought I'd give it to Emily, the little girl next door. They are so poor and have little money for extras."

"What a nice thing to do. You have always been a good-hearted person, Jen. I wish we had more money so we could do things like that more often."

Hai speaks up. "Jen feels good about her purchase and her plans to give it away. Anything that makes a person feel badly about himself is emotional abuse. We have just seen two scenes, the first in which the daughter has emotionally abandoned her father. She does not care how her father feels and has a complete lack of empathy for him."

"The second scene illustrated emotional abuse by domination. Treating her sister as a child, telling her how she should spend her money, making her feel inferior, or making her feel she (the sister) is always right, is another form of emotional abuse."

He looked around the room and asked, "Are there any questions?"

"What kind of person abuses others like this?" asked Dale Dobson, the attorney from Group Eight.

"Good question, Dale. Reading over the literature I found a rundown of an emotionally abusive person. He is usually very touchy when it comes to *others* making fun of *him* or making any kind of comment that shows a lack of respect. He may have difficulty apologizing and is always making excuses for his behavior and tends to blame others or circumstances for his own faults and blunders. He calls people and things names, often giving them labels. This person probably doesn't like himself and has many issues from his childhood that he has not worked out. He may even have been abused as a child and has not succeeded in working out his feelings of shame or guilt. There may be a rage inside him that he cannot control."

"Thank you for asking that question, Dale. Are there any others?"

Satisfied there were no questions, Hai said, "Today we have a film from Terra Nova Films produced by the Elder Abuse Institute of Maine. The title is **Martha's Story: A Lifetime of Walking on Eggshells**. Like the video last week, this is another story of spousal abuse."

The class was silent as the short fifteen-minute video began. It was the story of Martha, married to Jim for over fifty-one years. During that time he emotionally abused her, each time progressively worse. He browbeat her until she was always apprehensive, never knowing the right thing to do or say. She denied the abuse he heaped on her to herself and others, until finally she could take it no longer and reached out for help. Martha shares in her own words, memories about the abuse and how she was finally able to escape her situation."

"Are there any questions of the video?" asked Hai. There were none, so he continued. "Many times elderly abuse is caused by a spouse. The couple, like the one in the film, may have been married for years. The abuse gets worse until the partner is completely intimidated by the spouse. This type of abuse is called 'Domestic Abuse'. Sometimes the abuse begins in old age. The marriage may have been strained over the years, and with the coming of age, it just breaks down and abuse, by one or the other, begins. The majority of this type of abuse, however, is committed by men."

"What are some of the symptoms of elderly domestic emotional abuse?" Answering his own question he said, "The victims of such abuse may experience chaos, confusion, panic, and/or detachment. There may be a lot of friction while the abuse is taking place, and later, regret and confession on the part of the offender."

"These symptoms are more for domestic violence. How about emotional abuse by a caregiver or family member?" asked Marion Mahoney.

"Yes, good question," Hai responded. "There are other signs displayed by the victim such as:"

- Victim avoids eye contact with others and appears upset, scared, or despondent.
- Victim seems anxious, depressed, or withdrawn.
- Victim experiences sudden changes in eating or moods.
- Caregiver does not allow other people to call or visit the victim.
- Victim is not allowed by caregiver to make his own decisions.

"What are the characteristics of the elderly who are potential victims of emotional abuse?" asked Maria Delgado from Group Three.

"Good question. The following are some of the

characteristics, but not all victims suffer from them. Here are a few." Turning the page on the chart he had listed two items:

- Most victims are over 75 years old, and may have learning or memory problems or a long-term condition, such as dementia, diabetes, paralysis, or have suffered a stroke.
- The victim may have no relatives or friends who can take care of him and has difficulty getting along with others."

"The caregiver may also have some issues of his own." Turning the page on the chart he has listed caregiver issues:

- He may not have any money to speak of and depends on the victim for everything, including housing.
- He may drink excessively or be addicted to drugs.
- He may have a personality disorder, depression, or other mental illness.
- He may have a history of physical or sexual abuse.
- He may feel extreme stress taking care of the elder.

"An elderly person who suffers from emotional abuse may develop serious health problems including deep depression. Are there any more questions?"

Being none, Hai motioned to Emma that they were finished and they returned to their seats.

"Good job, Group Four. Excellent presentation. Let's take a short break and when we return Group Three will present on financial abuse."

LAUREL HALL

*"Gold is a fool's curtain,
which hides all his defects
from the world."*
Owen Feltham

Chapter Ten
Financial Abuse

After ten minutes or so the class was reseated. Emma, standing at the front of the room asked, "Are you ready, Group Three?"

"We are." Dr. Herman Sparks led the group followed by Dr. Maarten Johansen and the three nurses, Hugo Gonzales, Muriel Burns, and Maria Delgado. There was a round table at the front of the room and all the students seated themselves.

"We decided to give our presentation as a round table discussion," said Dr. Sparks beginning the discussion. "As people grow older they may experience short-term as well as long-term memory loss. If an elderly person has no family or friends and does not visit his doctor regularly, these symptoms may go unnoticed. Everyone needs human contact. Also, once an elderly person loses the right to drive and can no longer leave home, he is shut off from the world. Maria, do you have any information on this?"

"Yes," she replied. "Without human interaction, anyone can become susceptible to salesmen of all kinds, including telemarketers. These culprits look upon the elderly as fair game, as an opportunity to make money for themselves. A lonely person becomes more susceptible to excessive pressure and exploitation. This is especially true if diminished mental capacity is involved. They believe too easily the lies others tell them, and the trickery relatives may use to get the elder to sign documents handing over their property. Many times an elder won't even remember signing it."

"Sometimes neighbors may notice something peculiar going on," added Muriel, "but are afraid to get involved. They are afraid of 'butting in', getting involved in something that is none of their business and may get them in trouble with the family."

Dr. Johansen said, "Financial abuse is one of the most widespread forms of abuse, and the least expected. Does anyone have any knowledge of the methods used by the perpetrators?"

Dr. Sparks noted, "In some cases the victim has given someone full or partial access to his personal financial accounts and then, that person steals money from them."

Then Maarten added, "In other cases family members who hope to inherit money when the elder dies, may talk the victim into giving them some money now by assigning ownership of property to them or paying large amounts for something the offender desires. Such a person may sometimes turn the elder against other members of the family in an attempt to influence the will. The offender may also steal valuables or cash from the victim's home when they are sleeping or distracted. In some cases they have the elder put themselves (the offender) as manager of the victim's trust or to change the will so that they (the perpetrator) become one of the beneficiaries."

"Financial elder abuse is not always caused by family members. Sometimes it can be con-artists or thieves seeing an easy target. In some cases these perps are the caregivers of the elder, added Maria."

Dr. Mahoney asked, "How does one know this abuse is occurring?"

Muriel replied, "There are several indicators. For example, the elder's bills are not being paid. The caregiver may not allow the elder to see other relatives. Sometimes a relative may become overly interested in the elder's finances. It takes someone who loves the victim and watches their behavior to notice something is not just right and put a stop to it. Elderly people are often too weak both mentally and physically to take matters into their own hands. Getting in touch with an attorney may be just too much for the elder to do."

"That's right, Muriel," added Dr. Sparks. "Filing a lawsuit to recover damages from those involved in the financial abuse is only sometimes successful. Victims *may* be able to recover financial loss or property and money paid for a lawyer *may* be regained. Sometimes even punitive damages, but that is rare."

Dr. Johansen continued. "Financial abuse against the elderly can be stopped once it has been recognized as occurring. Most states have someone to investigate cases in which it has been determined an elder is unable to handle his finances properly. Does one of the attorneys in the class know the procedure as to how people can get help?" he asked.

Counselor Dobson stood up. "These people fall under the Adult Protective Services (APS). It usually goes like this. Once a complaint has been made, a worker will be sent to the home of the elder, conduct an interview, observe living conditions, and then report to another agency. If the APS deems financial abuse is occurring, it will make a referral to the District Attorney's Office. The APS will usually file a report to the local police, who also will refer it to the District Attorney. If there is enough evidence to prove a claim of elder financial abuse, then a criminal complaint can be filed against the offender. Additionally, elder law attorneys can get involved and file civil lawsuits to stop any further abuse and to recover money or property that was wrongfully taken."

"Thank you, counselor," said Dr. Johansen. "Are there any questions of Mr. Dobson?" There were none.

Emma walked to the front of the class. "Great presentation, Group Three." Picking up the bowl with the group numbers she selected two small pieces of paper. "Next week Group One will present on sexual abuse followed by Group Five, who will present on neglect and self-neglect. Have a good week, all."

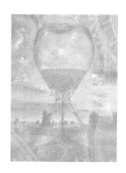

"I regard that man as lost,
Who has lost his sense of shame."
Plautus

Chapter Eleven
Sexual Abuse

I t had been a long hot week. It was hard to believe it was August already. The grass was turning brown and due to the drought many of the trees were stressed, some losing their leaves. Emma hopped into her car and drove to the hospital, where she took the elevator to the top floor. She was the first one there. She stared out the windows looking at the mountains. Some still had snow on their peaks. It was a beautiful setting. Slowly the students entered the room. Before long they were all seated. Emma enjoyed the class and the students and felt a bond with them that many teachers never have. She recalled a trigonometry class she had once taught. The students in that class bonded with her and each other like no other class she'd had before. Teaching them had been fun, a true joy.

"Good morning, everyone. I hope you had a great week. Today, Group One will give a presentation on elder sexual abuse. Are you ready, Group One?"

"We are" said Mike Benson, the policeman. He was dressed in full uniform and led the group to the front of the classroom followed by Dr. Robert Holland, Dr. Ricardo Gutierrez, and two nurses Barbara Edwards and Sally Calitri.

Robert Holland began. "We also decided to have a round table discussion format." Continuing, he said, I found the following definition. *Sexual abuse is any form of physical contact of a sexual nature with a person who lacks the mental capacity to give consent.* This includes rape, molestation, and even conversation of a sexual nature that the elder does not desire. Those responsible for this kind of abuse can include family members including the spouse, employees at a care facility such as a nursing home, and others. Sometimes one resident of a facility will assault another resident of the same facility. Barbara, I believe you plan to speak on the signs and symptoms of sexual abuse."

"Yes, I do." She began. "Some signs of sexual abuse may include physical injuries such as bruises, trouble walking or sitting, ripped, discolored, or bloody underwear, and maybe even contraction of a sexually transmitted disease they did not have prior to admittance to the facility. Another sign may be the manner in which the victim and abuser interact with each other. Does the victim appear to be afraid of that person?"

Officer Benson spoke next. "According to the National

Institute of Justice (NIJ), sexual abuse is one of the most understudied aspects of elder mistreatment. In a sponsored study on elder sexual abuse by the NIJ, they found the following:

- Psychological evaluation of elderly victims of sexual assault was rarely performed, and the older the victim, the less likelihood the offender would be convicted.
- If the victim displayed signs of physical pain and suffering, the offender was more likely to be charged with a crime.
- The likelihood of charges being brought against the assailant was slim if the victim lived in an assisted living facility."

"Dr. Gutierrez, what did you find?"

Ricardo looked at his papers and began: "In one state study on the sexual assault of those over 60, the following was found:

- Less than 35% of sexual assault victims over 65 reported their assault to the police. Sexual assault victims were six times more likely to be female.
- In another study over three years, it was found that frequently there was at least one witness to the abuse.
- In a three year study it was found the majority of sexual abuse cases occurred in a nursing home or other adult care facility.
- In yet another study it was determined most of the offenders were caregivers, followed by family members. These victims did not live in an institutional environment."

"Another study of older rape victims found that:

- Those attacked by strangers occurred most often in the victim's home, and a very small percentage of them reported the attack to the police.
- In about one third of rapes of older women, injuries were severe enough to require surgery."

As soon as Dr. Gutierrez had finished Sally Calitri stood up. "We have a video for you today from Terra Nova Films. The title of this film is *He Wouldn't Turn Me Loose:* **The Sexual Assault Case of 96-Year-Old Miss Mary** produced by: *National Clearinghouse on Abuse in Later Life & Terra Nova Films, Inc.*"

Marcie walked to the windows to close the shades. As soon as the room was darkened, Sally began the movie. The video was the real-life story of a ninety-six year-old woman called Miss Mary, who was financially abused by her grandson during the five years she lived with him and his wife. One evening when the grandson's wife was out, the grandson sexually abused Miss Mary for several hours, leaving her bruised from head to toe.

Once she was able to get help, Miss Mary was placed in a nursing home. Her family refused to believe her allegations and never visited her. Her only social contacts were with the staff and other residents of the nursing home.

Various professionals involved in the case helped her with her testimony and her grandson was successfully prosecuted.

After the video Sally continued. "One doesn't normally think of elderly sexual abuse, but it does exist and the consequences are devastating. These victims feel vulnerable to future abuse and don't know how to find safety. Worse, the abuser may be the caregiver, from whom there may be no escape. The victim may be embarrassed and ashamed, and as a result of the attack, may become depressed and detached."

Does anyone have any questions?" There were not any and the group returned to their places.

Emma stood in front of the class again. "Thank you all. Excellent presentation. Let's take a short break and then Group Five will present on neglect and self-neglect."

LAUREL HALL

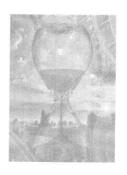

"In persons grafted in a serious trust,
Negligence is a crime."
Shakespeare

Chapter Twelve
Neglect and Self-neglect

Something had been troubling Emma ever since she started preparing for this course months ago. It was the dismay she felt as she studied problems suffered by the elderly and the fact that all of us are heading down the same road, some sooner than others. Thinking to herself she thought, *today I will discuss my feelings with the class and see if others share these same feelings.*

When all the students were reseated she began. "Group Five is to present today on neglect and self-neglect, but before they begin, I would like to share some of my personal feelings with you and perhaps, you will share some of yours with me."

"I have been feeling quite disheartened as I have learned about the fate of some of our senior citizens, realizing that we are all headed in the same direction - towards our journey's end. Some of you, like me, have more days behind you than in front, but for others your whole life is in front of you, unless of course, you hit a landmine. I have watched programs on television which show an actor dressing as an old man or old woman walking down the streets of a large city and how badly they were treated by the public. Many of these actors were dressed in ragged clothing and pretended to be homeless, pushing a store cart with all their 'belongings'. I saw how some of them were disrespected and abused. I found it all so depressing. And, from what I have learned, it doesn't matter if you are rich or poor, abuse can strike anyone. Have any of you felt the same way?"

Dr. Arthur raised his hand and began to speak. "I have seen my mother through several phases of her life – knowing her as a mother to me and my siblings, the conversations we shared, the fun we had as a family, watching her as a grandmother to my children. Now, I see the results of Alzheimer's disease. It is sad and discouraging and I wonder if that is what is in store for me. So, yes, it is depressing."

Nurse Hai Wong spoke next. "Growing old, losing your friends, your family, and those you love is difficult to think about. As a young person it is troublesome to conceive - we think ourselves immortal - but for most of us, that is our future. We will grow old and we will die."

Lucy stood up next. "I used to think old people didn't have the same feelings as we young ones do. I know now that is not true. Only their bodies grow old. As our body ages, it doesn't function as well as when it was new, but that doesn't mean we don't find humor in life, or love, or long for human touch.

THE SUNSET YEARS

Hopefully I have gained a little knowledge on how to grow old, how to care for my body. It's sad to think that as my body ages, my worth or value as a person may decline in the eyes of others. Because my youth is gone along with any beauty I might have had, some might think I was never young.   This class has given me a new look on the elderly and I believe new insights on aging. I hope sometime, we as a class, could discuss what we can do for ourselves, to help us face what is to be."

"Good idea," Emma added. "Perhaps we each can think on this and share our thoughts, possibly on the last day of class." The class nodded in agreement. "Thank you for sharing your thoughts with me. I do believe it is time for Group Five to give their presentation. Are you ready?"

"We are," they responded.

As Emma walked to the back of the room, Group Five came forward. Five nurses comprised the group - (Ann Haver, Mark Kellogg, Judy Kelp, Claire Donahue, and Barbara Kelly). They had decided to give their presentation in a round table discussion format.

Barbara, acting as leader, began.   "As people age they usually become weak and unable to defend themselves against abuse of any kind. Some may have partial or complete hearing loss, faded vision, and may not think as clearly as they once did. Some are dependent on another to care for them, much as a baby depends on his mother for his care. Failure of a caregiver to meet his responsibilities in caring for the elderly is neglect. Ann, can you tell us a little about neglect, please?"

Ann looked at her notes and began to speak. "Neglect can be either physical or emotional and includes such things as not providing food, medicine, heat, cooling fans or even assistance with daily activities of life that the older person cannot do for himself. It also includes lack of basic emotional support, respect, or love. For example, ignoring sobs, moans, or calls for help; keeping a person from having visitors; lack of support in doing stimulating activities such as going out for social or intellectual events".

"Good job, Ann. What can you add, Claire?"

"I read that neglect makes up over half of all reported cases of elder abuse and can be intentional or unintentional based on factors such as lack of knowledge or refusing to believe the elder needs as much care as he or she does. In plain English it means failing to pay attention to an elder, failing to care for them. Many elders that are abused are abused in their own home, as well as in facilities that are responsible for their care. This is happening not just in the United States but all around the world."

"I'm glad you brought that up, Claire. Many Americans feel other countries treat their elder citizens better than we do, but that's not true. Elder abuse is a global problem."

"Mark, what did you find out about the legal duties of a caregiver?"

"Well, I read that when an elderly person lives in a nursing home or other facility, that service has a legal duty to provide bedding, food, medication, and assistance with daily tasks along with stimulating activities. When the elder person lives with a family member or relative, their legal duty for caring for the older person is more difficult to define because there are no laws that lay out responsibilities for families specifically. However, if a caregiver is responsible for the elder, as is an institution, and fails to provide for him with the care a reasonable person would have provided, it can be considered unlawful elder neglect. States are beginning to pass laws that define the crime of elder neglect as well as other types of elder abuse. These laws vary widely in their definitions and effects."

"Very good, Mark. What did you find with regards to signs of elder neglect, Judy?"

"There are both physical and behavioral sign of neglect. Physical signs include unusual weight loss, skin sores, and unsanitary living conditions, improperly dressed for the weather and more. Behavioral signs can include crying, depression, difficulty sleeping, loss of appetite, emotionally withdrawn or detached, exhibiting fear toward the caregiver, confusion, and others."

"Being a caregiver for an elderly person is a full time job," said Barbara. "The caregiver needs to take care of himself as well. One thing he can do is to ask for help, get someone to come in and take care of the elder while he catches a break. Another thing is to find an adult daycare center for the patient. It is important that the caregiver stay healthy. Finding a support group for caregivers might be beneficial. If the caregiver becomes depressed over the situation, he should get counseling."

Lucy raised her hand. "What can we do to protect ourselves before we become elderly?"

The class laughed at the question, but in a nice way. "Good question, Lucy," Barbara said. "This list might help." She walked over to the large paper chart and flipped over the first page. There she had listed things individuals could do for themselves.

- Make sure your financial affairs are in order. Have you made your will?
- Stay in touch with your family. Don't become a loner, isolating yourself from humanity.
- Develop friendships.
- Consider volunteer work, for example, your local

hospital.

- Get active in senior centers, church functions, and the like.
- Know your neighbors.
- Have regular medical and dental appointments.
- Make sure someone is aware of your health status.

Then she added, "If and when the time comes and you are in a nursing home or under the care of someone, if you are unhappy with the care you are receiving and you feel you are being abused, tell someone you trust. Ask that person to report the abuse to the long-term care ombudsman in your area. That person would be found under the Adult Protective Services. Also, if you have to put your parents in a nursing home or assisted living facility, be sure to tell them also. Older people are afraid of rocking the boat."

"The second part of our presentation deals with self-neglect and all its implications," said Barbara. "Ann, could you tell us what you learned about the subject, please?"

"I read that self-neglect is when an older person intentionally does things that puts his health and safety or well-being in danger. Such behaviors might include not eating properly, not wearing clothing fitting for the weather, poor personal hygiene, not taking medication, dirty living conditions, and more. This is also known as self-abuse."

Continuing, she said, "Sometimes an elder person is not mentally competent to live alone. Other times the elder is mentally competent but chooses not to provide adequate care for himself. Generally, people are allowed to make bad choices, but in the case of an elderly person it begs the question: Do the elderly have less personal freedom to make life choices because of their age? It can be difficult to know if one should get involved."

Claire added: "Most elders who do neglect themselves are usually women who live alone. They are usually unhappy, depressed, and frail and may not have enough food, water, or heat. Their homes may be filthy and in need of major repairs. If they have pets, there may be feces about the house. They themselves may be unclean with dirty hair, nails, skin, and smell of urine. In addition they may have skin conditions as well as assorted physical needs. This includes such items as dentures, eye glasses, walkers, and such. They may have dementia and lack any interest in life. These just name a few."

"Barbara, did you find a video?" asked Claire.

"Yes, I found a video from Terra Nova Films, produced by the National Film Board of Canada. It is a video on Self-Neglect and asks some interesting questions. It's entitled **Mr. Nobody**."

Marcie walked to the windows and closed the shades.

Barbara continued. "**Mr. Nobody** is a Video which explores self-neglect and asks several important questions."

- "Do mentally capable seniors have the right to neglect themselves and their environs to the extent that they endanger themselves and/or offend the community?
- Do government agencies have the right to intervene?
- What should be done when antisocial or bizarre seniors refuse help?"

The room became quiet and the video began. **Mr. Nobody** was the story of 65-year-old Jack Huggins. Jack, a bachelor, had lived alone in his family's house ever since the death of his parents. He had many cats, on which he showered all his attention. The house was a mess, crammed with discarded appliances he had collected from curbside garbage.

When his neighbors complained to the Health Department about the condition of his home, Jack's troubles began. Health officials came and carted away his 'junk'. For a time, he was classified as incompetent and a state-appointed trustee monitored his financial affairs. Jack deeply resented this interference, having always functioned independently. "I never owed a person a cent and now I'm being treated like Mr. Nobody," he protested. Finally, a senior advocacy agency had him re-assessed by a psychiatrist.

Marcie reopened the shades. Barbara asked, "Does Jack have a right to neglect himself if he's hurting no one? Should the government intervene? If he doesn't want help, should help be forced on him? I don't know the answers to these questions, but they are food for thought."

Barbara added: "Social services cannot be everywhere. Family and friends are needed to help. What can one do? I think the following is a start.

- Become familiar with the signs of self-neglect.
- Telephone and/or visit the person. Volunteer to drive them somewhere. Help reduce the sense of aloneness the elder feels.
- When talking with the elderly person allow them to express themselves.
- Let the individual know it's okay to accept help from others.
- Contact APS if you feel the elder is self-neglecting."

Barbara closed the presentation with: "Growing old can be tough, and the longer you live, the tougher it can be.

Personally, I feel the emotional aspect of growing old is the most challenging. There's nothing you can do about it. So, our advice to you, prepare today for that tomorrow."

"Good presentation, Barbara, and all of you in Group Five."

Selecting two more pieces of paper from "the bowl" Emma said, "Next week Group Seven will present on abandonment followed by Group Six on institutional abuse. Have a good week."

LAUREL HALL

Alone, on a wide, wide sea,
So lonely t'was, that God himself
Scarce seemed there to be."
S. T. Coleridge

Chapter Thirteen
Abandonment

The week had sped by quickly. Emma and Jon had taken another trip to the mountains to relax, enjoy the scenery, and help reduce the stress Emma was feeling. *Fall is coming. I can feel it in the air,* she thought to herself. It was hard to believe that September was just around the corner. She remembered it seemed like the day after Labor Day the temperature had dipped right into fall. Emma liked that time of year. She remembered when their first grandchild was born in mid-September in Colorado; it had snowed. Coming from Texas seeing the white flakes falling gently to the ground had been thrilling to them.

Arriving at the classroom Emma saw several students already there. Among them were counselor Walter Carbonera, Marcie, and others. "Thank you for making this class possible," Walter said to Emma.

"Thank you for coming and becoming part of this class," she replied.

"Good job, Emma," said Marcie. "You have been the perfect teacher. I think all the students have enjoyed the classes and what they have learned. I also believe they have enjoyed the hands-on style of learning."

"Thank you, Marcie. I've enjoyed it, too. I must admit I was a bit intimidated at first."

Within a few minutes the class was seated. "Today Group Seven will present to us on Abandonment. Are you ready?"

"We are," they replied and the five members walked to the front of the class. In this group there were two doctors, Dr. Tom Parsons and Dr. Jim Howard, and three nurses, Janet Odom, Tina Hollis, and Irma Brown. Dr. Parsons spoke first. "In today's society seniors are discarded for both monetary and social reasons. This action leads to the decline of health, both physically and mentally. If a person has assumed the responsibility for an elderly person and then deserts him, that person can be prosecuted with criminal charges. Irma, what reasons did you find for people abandoning their elders?"

Irma replied, "I found that adult children abandon their elderly parents for many reasons. Here are a few."

- "Some children feel their fathers and mothers were terrible parents. Maybe this was due to mental or physical illness that may have impacted them during those years.

- Maybe their parents were alcoholics or addicted to drugs forcing their children, now adults, to care for them.
- Their parents today, as elders, are dominating and do not allow their children to assume responsibilities as adults.
- Their parents may have been abusive or neglectful of their children. Now adults, these children may hold grudges against their parents for the trauma they suffered as children and cannot forgive or forget the events of their childhood.
- Their parents may have only provided physical care, but were not emotionally caring. The needs of the parent came first over the needs of the child.
- Some parents are fiercely independent and refuse the care or advice of their children.
- Some adults just don't like their parents."

"I also read when people don't like their parents they feel no responsibility for caring for them. Also, in our country where there are social services to take care of 'abandoned parents', the effects of neglect may not be that obvious."

"Tina, how are seniors abandoned?"

"I read that when some seniors are placed in a nursing home facility, hospital, or some similar service very few people come to visit. Family members feel they have done their job by putting them there and now it is the facility's problem to care for them. This is especially true when family members don't like each other or their parents."

"Sometimes, the elderly person is taken to a shopping mall just to get them outside. Those taking them there find a bench for him/her to sit on and then leave them to go shopping, for how long we don't know. This, too, is considered abandonment."

"Janet, what can people do to help elderly relatives, parents and friends in their lives?" asked Dr. Howard.

"If a family lives out of the area, they can send weekly letters, telephone, and email."

"That's true, Janet. But what if a person has been alienated from his parents and now has to deal with them in their old age it can be more of a challenge. What happens then? Tom?"

"One thing a person in that situation could try is to find something they have in common to allow for conversation. It isn't easy. Don't bring up painful memories. Try to respect them as individuals. You, too, will be old someday. How do you want to be treated?"

"Good ideas," said Howard. "What about the caregiver? How can he/she get help? Irma?"

"Perhaps he can find a support group for himself. Being a caregiver can be challenging especially if there was a fractured relationship in the past. If there are siblings, perhaps responsibilities can be parceled out, giving each sibling a break now and then."

Walter Carbonera stood up to comment. "Anyone, friend, neighbor, or relative can call the Adult Protective Services if they feel an elderly person is being abandoned. APS is found in all states and will conduct a home visit and make an evaluation as to whether further investigation is warranted or if protective services are needed. If that is the case, police will be called in to further investigate the situation."

"Does anyone have any questions or comments?" asked Dr. Parsons.

Muriel raised her hand. "Is APS also in Guam, the District of Columbia, and the US Virgin Islands?"

"Yes, it is," Dr. Parsons replied. "Any other questions?" Being none, the group sat down. "Good report," said Emma. "Let's take a short break, and then Group Six will give their presentation.

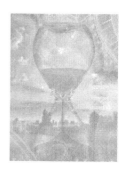

*"Institutional Abuse of Older People
is common, insidious, and
a serious indictment
of the caring professions,
including medicine".*

Lucy Alexander

Chapter Fourteen
Institutional Abuse

T he class was milling about, visiting with each other and munching on the goodies provided. It had rained for the last three days on and off giving the grass and trees some much-needed water, but today the humidity was a bit high, especially for Colorado. No one was complaining. Everyone was happy with the rain. Soon all the students were reseated. "Group Six, I believe you are presenting today on

Institutional abuse. Are you ready?"

"We are," they said and walked to the front of the class. Group Six had two nurses, Jamie Luciano and Bethany Rolf; Dr. Evans, the hospital doctor; and two x-ray technicians, Jeanne Levine and Sarah Driscoll.

Dr. Evans began the presentation. "We will also do a round table discussion type format. Institutional elder abuse is a disgraceful act committed upon older individuals who are unable to protect themselves. What makes this abuse so outrageous is that the family has paid good money to the very people or facility that is abusing their loved one. Such abuse can have a severe effect on the quality of life of the elderly individual. Sometimes the staff must follow certain procedures and routines and those become more important than the residents. When staff becomes frustrated abuse is likely to happen. There may be cases where one staff member has too many patients to care for properly. During this session we will discuss what you should look for to identify that abuse is occurring in a nursing home."

"Jeanne, what did you find out about signs of institutional abuse?"

"There are a number of signs of general neglect and elder abuse. Walking into a nursing facility a good indication of poor care may be an overpowering smell of urine, especially if it never goes away. If someone you are visiting in a nursing home has any of the following - skin sores or a rash on his/her body, noticeable hunger, or severe thirst - these can all be indications of institutional abuse. In addition, if their clothing is dirty, their bed linens unchanged and smelly, or their living quarters dusty and dirty, these can be signs of neglect as well."

"Jamie, what did you find to be signs of institutional physical abuse?"

"There are many signs of physical abuse such as bruises, swellings, or discoloration on the face or body. The resident may be afraid of a particular employee or may hesitate to explain certain wounds or bruises."

Bethany spoke next. "Americans are living longer than ever before. Better health care and programs such as Social Security, Medicare, pension plans and/or annuities allow most senior citizens to lead a fairly good life. The nursing home business has blossomed and approximately a million and a half older Americans reside in one. However, corruption, neglect, and abuse occur within the business, and many facilities provide unsatisfactory care for their residents. There has also been a large increase in the occurrence of elderly abuse."

Sarah spoke next. "I read about laws, rules and regulations. Both federal and state governments have created laws, rules, and regulations and have established a 'Bill of Rights' for residents living in nursing homes. Failure to follow these rules can cause a facility to lose their Medicare or Medicaid certification, which, in turn, denies them federal reimbursements. In addition, federal and state inspectors are also able to levy fines on nursing homes that do not follow these guidelines. This has been somewhat successful in keeping these facilities in check, but has come nowhere close to the desired goal of eliminating institutional abuse of the elderly."

"Depending upon the state in which you live, there are laws that allow you to bring a claim against a nursing home or facility for violating a resident's rights. In some states reporting elderly abuse in nursing homes is mandatory. If specific persons or facilities do not report elderly abuse they may be found guilty of a misdemeanor offense. Certain states may also hold the home liable for damages to the injured resident."

Dr. Evans rose to speak. "If you feel that someone in a nursing home is suffering from abuse, here are some steps to take."

- "First, file a complaint with the state in which you live. State health agencies are required by law to investigate complaints of nursing home abuse. Go to the APS, the department of Social Services.
- The agency receiving the complaint will investigate the accusations. If the investigators find abuse or neglect, they will make provisions to help protect the victim. When making a complaint against a nursing home you should include the following:
- Address
- Telephone Number
- Email address
- Relationship to the victim
- The given name and any other name that the resident goes by.
- What condition prompted the elder to live in a nursing home
- A detailed account of the abuse by the nursing home. Include dates, time, and any other pertinent information you can give such as names of staff, shift, etc. Include any staff member you have spoken with about the abuse.
- If victim was taken to the emergency room, include medical records. Make and keep copies for yourself.
- If the victim dies, obtain a copy of the autopsy

and include it with the complaint."

"The grievance does not have to be complicated and long, but it must include all relevant data."

"The state agent handling the complaint should connect with the individual who filed the complaint within a few days to discuss it in more detail. He then usually makes a surprise visit to the facility to investigate the abuse complaint. In the case that the alleged offense is found to be true, the state will take whatever steps it feels are appropriate. It is advisable to send a copy of the complaint to the APE (Association for the Protection of the Elderly). They can be of great assistance to you. Next, hire an attorney to help you. Does anyone have any questions?"

"Exactly what do these facilities do to harm residents?" asked Tina.

"Sometimes, elderly residents in nursing facilities are left without food, water, or may lie in unclean bed linens. If a resident cannot reach the call button or has difficulty communicating with the staff, they are at more risk."

"Do any states consider abandonment a violation of law?" asked Lucy.

"In New Jersey, Pennsylvania, and California abandoning residents is a violation of law and trials may occur which can include financial settlements."

"Is there any website one can visit which will compare nursing homes?" asked Marcie.

"As a matter of fact, there is. If you go to Medicare.gov you can select a tab which compares nursing homes in your area. These homes are Medicare/Medicaid certified and are ranked one to five stars. This site will help individuals make an informed decision about nursing homes in their area."

"Are there any more questions?"

There were none. Dr. Evans beckoned to Emma that they

were finished and the group sat down.

"Good presentation," Emma said. "Congratulations to both groups for their presentations today. Next week is our last week of class." Taking the bowl there was only one piece of paper left. "Group Eight – you're on for next week. After their presentation we will have a discussion on our feelings on growing old and the problems of aging. Have a good week, all."

THE SUNSET YEARS

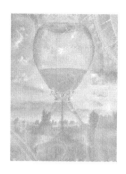

America did not invent human rights.
In a real sense...human rights invented America.

Fmr. President Jimmy Carter

Chapter Fifteen
Residents' Rights

J on and Emma were planning a trip to the Grand Canyon
and other nearby sites for late September. They had planned
to drive from their home and visit other places along the
way. As she drove to class Emma was pleased with the way the
class turned out. She had enjoyed her guest speakers and she
felt the students had done a terrific job on their presentations.
As she arrived at the sixth floor, a number of students were
already present. Within minutes the remainder arrived. One
thing that had impressed her was that not one student had

missed a class.

After greeting the students she walked to the front of the class. "Today Group Eight will present on Resident's Rights. Are you ready Group Eight?"

"We are" they replied. There was one doctor, Jacob Webber; two attorneys, Walter Carbonera and Dale Dobson; and two nurses, Betty Cornwell and Jane Ruth, in the group. Dr. Webber began the presentation. "When a person moves into a long-term health care facility they must be given a copy of their rights as a resident and they must understand them. If for some reason, usually medical, the person cannot understand these rights, those rights must be given to their guardian and the guardian must understand them completely. These rights were put in place in 1987 during the federal Nursing Home Reform Act. In addition to his rights as a citizen he also has rights that have been mandated by the federal and state governments known as the resident 'Bill of Rights'. Dale, would you discuss these rights?"

"I will. "Patients in a nursing home have many rights. These rights include:

- The Right to be Informed: They must also be given information about their finances, bills, and personal allowance. Residents are to be treated with respect and dignity. Abuse is illegal.
- The Right to Secure Possessions: Residents have the right to control their personal belongings and financial matters.
- Rights Regarding Transfers and Discharges: Resident must receive a 30-days' notice of being transferred or discharged. If being relocated to a different facility they must be provided with information about the new facility, and be given the opportunity to appeal the decision. The resident must be made aware of why he or she is

being transferred or discharged.

- The Right to Complain: If a resident feels he is not being treated properly, he has the right to complain without fear of reprisal.
- Rights Regarding Visitations: All residents have the right to speak promptly with their doctor, lawyer, or relatives. Relatives must be allowed to visit at any time unless a visitor is deemed a risk to the patient. Nursing home facilities must allow visitation rights with any state or federal agency that provides health, social, or legal services."

"In addition to patients' rights, nursing homes have duties and responsibilities to their residents. Betty, can you discuss those, please?" asked Walter.

"Yes, sir," she replied.

- "It is the responsibility of any nursing home to deliver quality care which includes keeping the patients healthy and clean, along with clean living quarters, and stimulating activities.
- Hiring and training qualified people to staff the facility is another important duty of any nursing home. Continuing education for its employees should be provided as well as annual training, which would include a review of the guidelines provided by the nursing home with regards to care and safety.
- The nursing home facility must provide a safe environment for its residents. This would include safety drills for weather or fire, handling spills, and the like.
- All residents must be treated with respect and dignity. Because most residents in a nursing home are unable to care for themselves and rely on the staff for help, the facility must follow HIPAA laws, and have patient's

properly clothed, groomed and presentable at all times.

- Nursing homes should hold joint meetings with all personnel that deal with patients about once a month. This would include their physician, pharmacist, nurses, social workers, and others to discuss and make changes to each patient's care plan."

"Jane, do you have anything to add?" asked Dr. Webber.

"Yes. I found there are many myths and realities of nursing homes with which most people are unaware.

- If a patient is on Medicaid he cannot get the same treatment as other residents who are not on Medicaid. This is simply not true. Medicaid patients must get the same services as anyone else.

- Another myth is that only the facility can decide what care the patient receives. Not so. Family and patient have the right to be involved in the treatment.

- The facility says it has no place for family members to gather. The home must provide a private space for family meetings.

- If a resident is difficult or refuses treatment he can be evicted. Not so. Those are not reasons to justify eviction.

- If the patient does not improve physically, treatment or therapy can be discontinued. Not so. Medicare may pay even if the patient does not improve."

Jane continued. "These are only a few. People interested in learning more about nursing home myths and realities only need to Google 'Nursing home myths and realities'. There they will find a wealth of information."

Walter Carbonera summed it up: "Any nursing home is a medical facility whose residents are usually unable to care for themselves and need supervised care around the clock. This is their home. It is the duty of the facility to provide quality care and meet the needs of all its patients by hiring qualified personnel and making the residence a safe place to live."

Emma walked to the front of the room clapping her hands in appreciation. "Thank you. Great job! Let's take a short break and when we come back we'll share our own ideas on growing old."

LAUREL HALL

THE SUNSET YEARS

..."If only when one heard
That Old Age was coming,
One could bolt the door,
Answer "not at home"
And refuse to meet him!"

Anonymous
Japanese Poem

Chapter Sixteen
Thoughts on Growing Old

Emma stood in front of the class. "For this last day, this last half of class we had decided to discuss our feelings on growing old. For me, leading this class has given me new insights on aging, aspects with which I was totally unfamiliar. I have learned much on dementia and Alzheimer's disease, senior issues and how to help seniors in dealing with the challenges they face. Although I am very familiar with child abuse and the effects it has on its victim's lives, I was completely blind when it came to elder abuse. This has been an eye opener for me. For the current elderly we can learn the signs of elder abuse, visit them, volunteer to help them and the like, but for us, how can we prepare ourselves for old age? Do any of you have any comments you would like share with the class?"

Marion Mahoney, from Group Three, stood. "I have never thought about growing old. But what choice do we have? I have learned it's important to take care of our body today so that it will serve us well as we age."

Dr. Parsons spoke next. "I believe it is very important to stay active as long as you can. Have a hobby, and of course, I always want to have a dog."

Sarah Driscoll from X-ray stood. "My husband and I have started talking about growing old and what we want to happen. We have begun an exercise program and watching our diet and keeping our bodies healthy."

Barbara Kelly, a nurse from Group Five, stood to speak. "I don't like the thought of growing old. I look at my mother, she's 94 and in great shape. Her sister is 97, also in great shape. And, if I were to ask them how they feel about being old, they would say they love it. But, I don't want to be old. Maybe I'm just afraid. I take care of my skin, that's important to me. But as someone said, what choice do I have?"

Dale Dobson, an attorney from Group Eight, spoke next. "Growing old is something I've never really given much thought. Few people talk about what they are going to do when they grow old. This class has given me food for thought. I think I will start watching what I eat, and perhaps do a few stretching exercises."

Mark, a nurse from Group Five, said, "I think people don't

want to talk about growing old, because what is left? Death! People don't want to talk about dying. As a nurse I have watched people die. Most of you in this room have as well. Death doesn't frighten me now, but I am curious about what comes after."

Rockey Evans, the hospital doctor from Group Six slowly stood. "I have done much thinking on aging since this course began. So many people assume that old age is when the body deteriorates, when reasoning abilities fail, when life is all but over. They fail to recognize what many seniors possess: energy, knowledge, time, vigor. No longer do they live in the future; they live in the 'now' and are able to do what they want to do, not what others want them to do. Avoiding landmines, taking care of our bodies so they serve us well as seniors, old age can be a good time of life. But we need to prepare for it wisely."

Gary Friend spoke next. "Sometimes as people age they get angry and are constantly complaining of their aches and pains. I would imagine they complained when they were younger as well. Then there are others who know it all, who think they are the experts on everything, and need to share it with everyone, especially their adult children. Younger people don't care to be around seniors that act this way. I think it is important to develop a positive attitude and accept your children as adults who have some knowledge about life."

Dr. Johansen stood. "I think we are missing something here, and that is money. Each of us needs to save for our retirement and old age. Without money, what we can do is limited. More than that, we may become a burden on others."

"I agree," said Susan Bonds, the OB nurse. "Having financial resources is very important, but equally important is good health. One is no good without the other."

"I think having a good sense of humor is also important," said Walter Carbonera. "No one wants to be around a grumpy old man or woman."

"I believe it is important to be up to date on what's going on in the world. Listen to the news and read magazines. Be able to have conversations on something other than our own aches and pains," added Dr. Arthur. "And, don't retire from living," he added.

Ann Haver, who had been sitting quietly, stood hesitantly as if questioning herself as to whether she should share her thoughts. A petite brunette, Ann had been quiet during most of the class, participating only during her group presentation. She was clearly nervous as she spoke. "During these past few weeks I have mulled over in my mind growing old and the end of the journey. It's been difficult for me because I don't like to think of death and dying. So, I have come up with this philosophy which I thought perhaps I would share with you. For me, I like to separate the body and the soul. By soul I mean the 'essence' that is me." Holding out her arm and pinching it, she said: "This piece of flesh doesn't represent who I am. I just live in it. The soul, the life that is me, that is ageless. I have come to believe only the body grows old and only the body dies. I find that comforting. I have learned in this class to take care of my body, to eat healthy, exercise, stay socially active and interested in what is going on in the world and to treasure my family and friends. That way I can enjoy this body to its fullest even as it grows old and weak."

"Wow! I like that, Ann," Emma replied. Thank you for sharing your philosophy."

"Are there any other remarks, comments, or observations?" There were none. Emma looked at the class and smiled. "The other day I was visiting with my ten year old grandson. He looked at me and said 'you are old, Nannie'. Yes, Hunter, I am old, I replied. Then I looked at him and asked: 'How do you feel about growing old?' He thought a minute, looked at me and replied, 'I'm not comfortable with it'. I laughed. 'That's all right' Hunter. You have years to adjust." The class laughed along with Emma."

Continuing, she said, "I believe we have come up with some good ideas. Let's see if we can summarize."

- We need to save for our retirement.
- We need to keep our bodies healthy by exercising and eating properly.
- Have a hobby.
- Stay current with news and what's going on in the world.
- Develop a positive attitude. Avoid complaining.
- Avoid being the expert on everything.
- Do not retire from living.
- Develop a sense of humor.
- Learn to live in the 'now'.
- Have a dog. They make wonderful companions.

Emma continued. "The other day I received this email from a friend. I don't know who wrote it, but it touched me and many others. I tried to discover the name of the author by googling the title, but could not find it. During my search, I found many other people were also impressed by his words." As she handed out a sheet of paper to each student, she said, "I thought you might appreciate it."

LAUREL HALL

AND THEN IT IS WINTER

"You know. . . time has a way of moving quickly and catching you unaware of the passing years. It seems just yesterday that I was young, just married and embarking on my new life with my mate. Yet in a way, it seems like eons ago, and I wonder where all the years went. I know that I lived them all. I have glimpses of how it was back then and of all my hopes and dreams."

"But, here it is... the 'back nine' of my life and it catches me by surprise...How did I get here so fast? Where did the years go and where did my youth go? I remember well seeing older people through the years and thinking that those older people were years away from me and that, 'I was only on the first hole' and the 'back nine' was so far off that I could not fathom it or imagine fully what it would be like."

"But, here it is...my friends are retired and getting gray...they move slower and I see an older person now. Some are in better and some worse shape than me...but, I see the great change...Not like the ones that I remember who were young and vibrant...but, like me, their age is beginning to show and we are now those older folks that we used to see and never thought we'd become. Each day now, I find that just getting a shower is a real target for the day! And taking a nap is not a treat anymore... it's mandatory! Cause if I don't on my own freewill... I just fall asleep where I sit!"

"And so...now I enter into this new season of my life unprepared for all the aches and pains and the loss of strength and ability to go and do things that I wish I had done but never did! But, at least I know, that though I'm on the 'back nine', and I'm not sure how long it will last... this I know, that when it's over on this earth...it's over. But I believe a new adventure will begin!"

"Yes, I have regrets. There are things I wish I hadn't done...things I should have done, but indeed, there are many things I'm happy to have done. It's all in a lifetime."

"So, if you're not on the 'back nine' yet...let me remind you that it will be here faster than you think. So, whatever you would like to accomplish in your life please do it quickly! Don't put things off too long! Life goes by quickly. So, do what you can today, as you can never be sure whether you're on the 'back nine' or not! You have no promise that you will see all the seasons of your life... so, live for today and say all the things that you want your loved ones to remember...and hope that they appreciate and love you for all the things that you have done for them in all the years past!"

"Life is a gift to you. The way you live your life is your gift to those who come after. Make it a fantastic one. And remember: *Today is the oldest you've ever been, yet the youngest you'll ever be, so enjoy this day while it lasts.*"

Author Unknown

"Emma, thank you for sharing this email," commented Jennifer Thomas. "I feel certain each of us is equally touched by this person's thoughts. I know I was."

"Thank you. I have so enjoyed getting to know each of you, of sharing information with you, learning together. It has truly been a privilege, one I will never forget. Thank you so very much for your graciousness and hospitality."

The students all stood and gave Emma a round of applause. Suddenly, it was over. Emma would miss these people she had come to know as students and friends.

Many of the students circled around Emma, giving her their own special thanks and hugs. Marcie walked to the front of the room. Putting her arms around Emma, she said, "For me this has been one of the best continuing education classes we have held. Thank you for taking the assignment."

"Marcie, it was my pleasure. Would you like to have coffee and brunch with me?"

"I would like that, Emma. Let's go."

About the Author

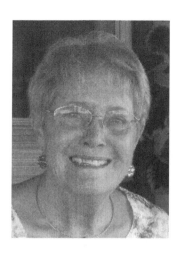

L aurel Hall, a retired teacher, was born and raised in New England. Once a resident of Texas for more than forty years, she currently lives in Colorado with her husband. *The Sunset Years* is her fourth book, written after a friend said to her, "I wish you had written on elder abuse."

She is the author of *Providence*, a memoir of the abuse she endured as a child and the impact it had on her life, *Betrayed, The Aftermath of Child Abuse*, on what happens to children that have been abused and do not receive help before they become adults, and *Expressions* (a book of illustrated poetry). You can learn more about Laurel Hall by visiting her website/blog http://www.thisnewdawn.com

Thank you for taking the time to read this book. If you would like to review it at the site of purchase, or to suggest it to others, I would be very grateful.   LH

THE SUNSET YEARS

References

AAA, Area Agencies on Aging, include older adult protective services. Their phone number for the local AAA offices can be found under the blue pages under Abuse/Assault.

Administration for Community Living ACL,
IOM Forum on Global Violence Prevention, http://
acl.gov/NewsRoom/Blog/2013/2013_05_02

Administration on Aging: Http://aoa.gov/AoARoot/
AoA_Programs/Elder_Rights/Legal/Index,
National Center on Elder Abuse, (Title II),
Administration on Aging: Long-Term Care Ombudsman Program,
(OAA, Title VII, Chapter 2, 711/712http://aoa.gov/
AoARoot/AoA_Programs/ Elder_Rights/Ombudsman)

Alzheimer's: Diabetes of the Brain?,
http://www.doctoroz.com/videos/alzheimers-diabetes-brainBy Dr.
Suzanne DeLaMonte Alpert Medical School, Brown University
Neuropathologist, Rhode Island Hospital, Posted on 4/06/2011

Alzheimer Prevention website:
http:// www.alzprevention.org/index.php
Alz.org, Alzheimer's associaltion, Music Therapy
http://www.alzfdn.org/EducationandCare/music therapy.html

Alzheimer's Foundation of America http://www.
alzfdn.org/EducationandCare/musictherapy.htmlc

Andrew Chadwick,Abandonment of Elderly Parents and Cultural
Values, Abandoning Elderly Parents: An analysis
Anthology of World Poetry, **An**, Halcyon House, NY

Aquariums May Pacify Alzheimer's Patients, study,
www.sciencedaily.com/releases/1999/07/990716071547.htm

Art and Music Therapy for Alzheimer's Disease
http://www.webmd.com/alzheimers/alzheimers- therapies-music-art-

more?page=2

American Music Therapy Association, http://
www.musictherapy.org/about/quotes/

Assisted Living Today http://assistedlivingtoday.
om/2012/03/music-and-dementia/

Brain Blogger.com Topics from Multidimensional Biopsychosocial
Perspective
Can Horses Help Dementia Patients? « Office of Geriatrics ...
ogg.osu.edu/can-**horses**-help-**dementia-patients**

Center for Elders and the Courts, The (CEC) serves as
a national resource center dedicated to serving courts
throughout the United States on issues related to aging,
probate, and elder abuse. The Center for Elders and the
Courts provides information on current legislation on
elder abuse in each state throughout the United States.
Crimes Against Older Adults Task Force, How to
Recognize   Emotional   Abuse,   http://crimes
againstolderadultsbucks.org/c_emotional-abuse.php
Denver Post The, Colorado advocates push mandatory
reporting law for elder abuse, Sara Burnett, 10/24/2011

E. Carlson, Twenty Common Nursing Home Problems and the Laws
to Resolve Them, *Clearinghouse Review Journal of Poverty Law and
Policy,* January/February 2006 39(9–10):519–33

eHow, Emotional Abuse in the Elderly, by Donna
McFadden, http//www. ehow. com/about_6372157_
emotional-abuse-elderly.html, 6/25/2013

FOOD FOR THE BRAIN, About dementia/Alzheimer's disease,
http://www.foodforthebrain.org/nutrition-solutions/dementia-and-
alzheimer%E2%80%99s-disease/about-dementiaalzheimer%E2%80%99s-
disease.aspx

GAO, Report to the Chairman, Special Committee on Aging, U.S.
Senate, March 2011. Elder Justice, Stronger Federal Leadership Could

Enhance National Response to Elder Abuse. GAO-11-208

Garner, J. and Evans, S. (2002) An Ethical Perspective on Institutional Abuse of Older Adults. The Psychiatrist 26, 164-166) Lucy Alexander

Helpguide.org, Lewy Body Dementia; Signs, Symptoms, Treatment, Caregiving; http://www. helpguide.org/elder/lewy_boy_disease.htm

Helpguide.org, Elder Abuse and Neglect, http://www. helpguide.org/mental/elder_abuse

Holt, Malcolm G. Elder Sexual Abuse in Britain: Preliminary Findings. Journal of Elder Abuse and Neglect. 5(2): 63-71. 1993.

How Animal Therapy Helps Dementia Patients - Alzheimer's ... www.everydayhealth.com/alzheimers/...therapy...patients.aspx

How Can Pets Benefit Alzheimer's Patients? www.**alzheimers**.net/2013-05-17/**alzheimers-pet-therapy**

Impact of Music Therapy on Language Functioning in Dementia The," University of Miami's School of Medicine in Florida., Dr. Ardash Kumar, M. Brotons and S.M. Kroger

Klaus, Patsy A. Crimes Against Persons Age 65 or Older, 1992-97. January 2000. U.S. Department of Justice. Bureau of Justice Statistics. http://www.ojp.usdoj.gov/bjs/pub/pdf/cpa6597.pdf

LiveStrong.com, What are the Duties of a Nursing Home, Julie Boehlke, Aug 16, 2013

Medicare.gov, Nursing Home Compare, The Official Government sight for Medicare

National Association of States United for Aging and Disabilities (NASUAD, Elder Rights Programs, http:// www.nasuad.org/tasc/elder_rights_   program.html)

National Committee for the Prevention of Elder Abuse The (NCPEA) http://www.ask.com/wiki/Elder_

abuse?o=3986&qsrc=999 - cite_note-33

Oregon Coalition against Domestic and Sexual Violence,
http://www.ocadsv.org/i-am-looking-help/elders

Parentgiving, the ultimate senior care resource,
http:// www.parentgiving.com/elder-care/music-as-a-tool-to-improve-communications-skills-in-alzheimers-patients/

Pennsylvania Coalition Against Rape (PCAR).
http://www.pcar.org

Pet Therapy for Alzheimer's Patients - The Health Benefits ...
www.applewoodourhouse.com/**pet-therapy-for-alzheimers**...

Pet Therapy: Animal Therapy For Alzheimers And Other Elderly
www.essortment.com/pet-therapy-animal-therapy-alzheimers
Ramsey-Klawsnik, Holly. Elder Sexual Abuse: Preliminary Findings. Journal of Elder Abuse and Neglect. 3(3): 73-90. 1991.

Rhode Island Hospital, The Alzheimer's Disease and Memory Disorders Center, Diet and Dementia: Toxic Preservatives Contribute to Alzheimer's Disease, Suzanne de la Monte, MD, ,
http://www.rhodeislandhospital.org/services/alzheimers/memory-disorders/diet-and-dementia-toxic-preservatives-contribute-to-alzheimers-disease.html

Self-Neglect, Washington State Dept of Social and Health Services; http://www.dshs.wa.gov/

SeniorsList, Seniors Most Concerning Issues; Shirley Cohen 6/25/2013

SeniorsList,Find Help for Elder Abuse

SeniorsList,Nursing Home Abuse and Neglect, by Marya Sieminski

SeniorsList, Emotional Abuse in Nursing Homes, by Hayes

SeniorsList, Signs of Nursing Home Abuse,
by Tara Pingle

SeniorsList,Nursing Home Abuse, by
George Dickerman

**SeniorsList, Home Care Agency; Assisted Living; Senior
Care**, Signs of Nursing Home Abuse, Tara Pingle 6/25/2013

SeniorsList, Your Source for Aging Well, www.seniorslist.com

**SeniorsList, Financial Abuse of the Elderly Can Go Unnoticed,
James Druman**, www.seniorslist.com **6/25/2013**

7 Stages of Alzheimer's & Symptoms | Alzheimer's Association
www.alz.org/alzheimers_disease_stages_of_alzheimers.asp

Sexual Abuse of Older Adults: Preliminary Findings
of Cases in Virginia. Journal of Elder Abuse and
Neglect. Teaster, Pamela, Roberto, Karen, Duke, Joy,
and Myeonghwan, Kim. 12(3/4): 1-16. 1993.
Takepart, http://www.takepart.com/article/2012/09/30/secret-
preventing-alzheimers-simple-skipping-processed-foods,Can Skipping
Processed Foods Prevent Alzheimer's?, September 30, 2012, _Andri
Antoniades_

Terra Nova Films, Inc.,9848 S. Winchester Ave., Chicago, IL,
60643, http//www.terraova.org, Phone: (773)881-8491

Warning Signs of Elder Abuse, University of Delaware
under a grant from The National Center on Elder Abuse.

Web MD, Dementia

Web MD, Alzheimer 's disease

Wikipedia.com, Music therapy

Wikipedia.com, Sundowning

WiseGEEK.com http://www.wisegeek.com/what-are- the-benefits-
of-music-therapy-for-alzheimers.htm

LAUREL HALL

THE SUNSET YEARS

CLASS ROSTER

Group 1: Sexual abuse
Mike Benson, officer
Robert Holland, Gastroenterologist
Barbara Edwards, Nurse
Sally Calitri, Nurse
Ricardo Gutierrez, ER doctor

Group 2: Physical abuse
Rebecca Rodriguez, Nurse
Gary Friend, MRI
Sharon Linn, Nurse
John Arthur, Surgeon
Marcie Withers, Hospital
Coordinator

Group 3: Financial abuse
Herman Sparks, Pathologist
Hugo Gonzales, Nurse
Muriel Burns, Nurse,
Maria Delgado, Nurse
Maarten Johansen, Orth. Surgeon

Group 4: Emotional abuse
Hai Wong, Nurse
Susan Bonds, Nurse
Lucy Rose, Lab
Jennifer Thomas, Internal Medicine
Marion Mahoney, Anesthesiologist

Group 5: Neglect abuse
Ann Haver, Nurse
Mark Kellogg, Nurse
Judy Kelp, Nurse
Claire Donahue, Nurse
Barbara Kelly, Nurse

Group 6: Institutional abuse
Jamie Luciano, Nurse
Bethany Rolf, Nurse
Rockey Evans, Hospital Doctor
Jeanne Levine, X-ray
Sarah Driscoll, X-ray

Group 7: Abandonment
Tom Parsons, Heart Specialist
Jim Howard, Pediatrician
Janet Odom, Nurse
Tim Hollis, Nurse
Irma Brown, Nurse

Group 8: Patient's Rights
Jacob Webber, Hematologist
Janet Ruth, Nurse
Betty Cornwall, Surgical Nurse
Dale Dobson, Civil Rights Attorney
Walter Carbonera, Attorney, Int'l
Law

LAUREL HALL

THE SUNSET YEARS

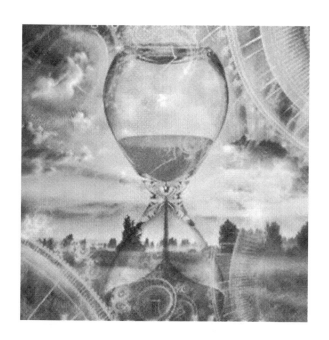

Made in the USA
Lexington, KY
09 December 2013